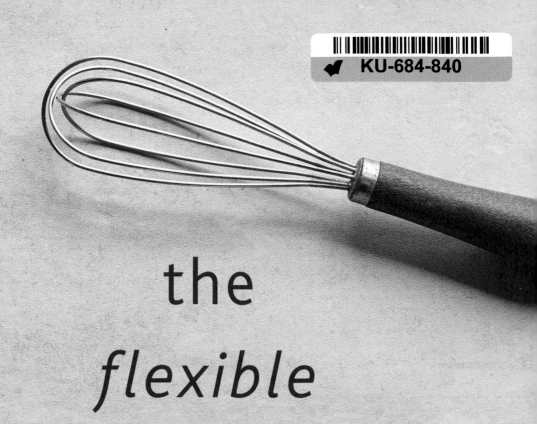

the *flexible* baker

JO PRATT

PHOTOGRAPHY BY MALOU BURGER

WHITE
LION
PUBLISHING

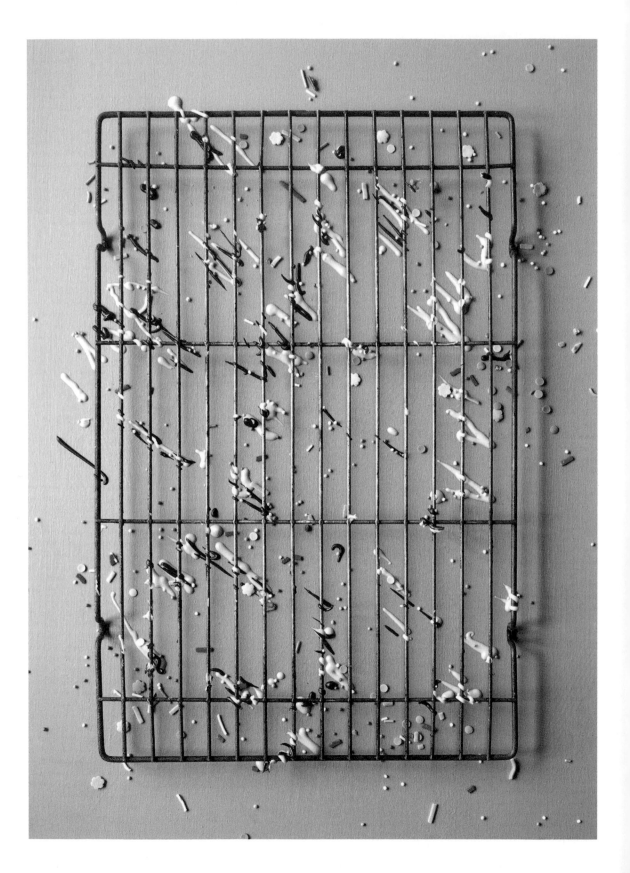

the
flexible
baker

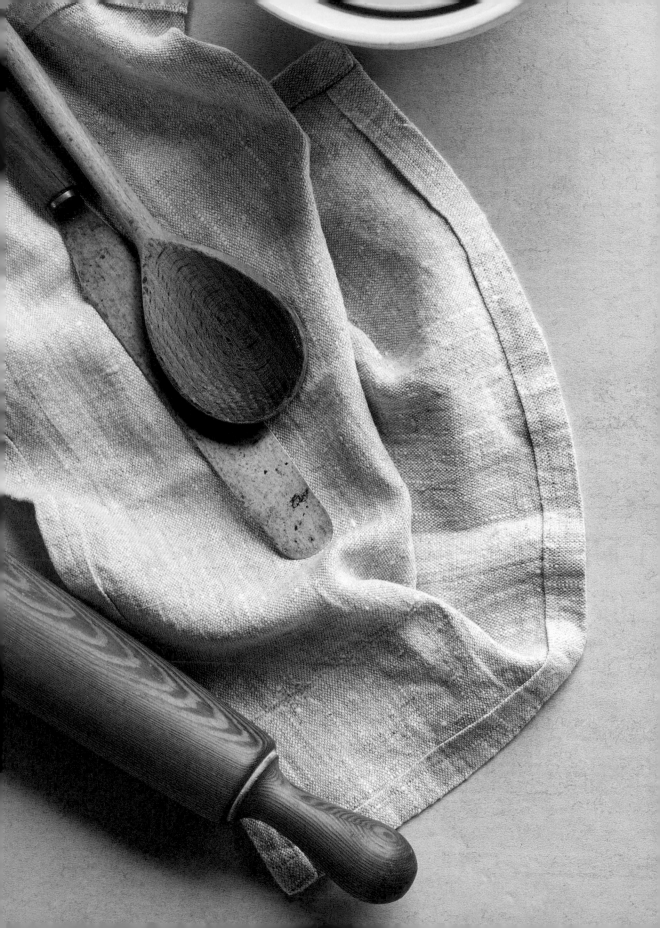

St. Helens Libraries

Please return / renew this item by the last date shown. Items may be renewed by phone and internet.

Telephone: (01744) 676954 or 677822
Email: libraries@sthelens.gov.uk
Online: sthelens.gov.uk/librarycatalogue

𝒯

2 5 AUG 2022

 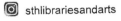

Contents

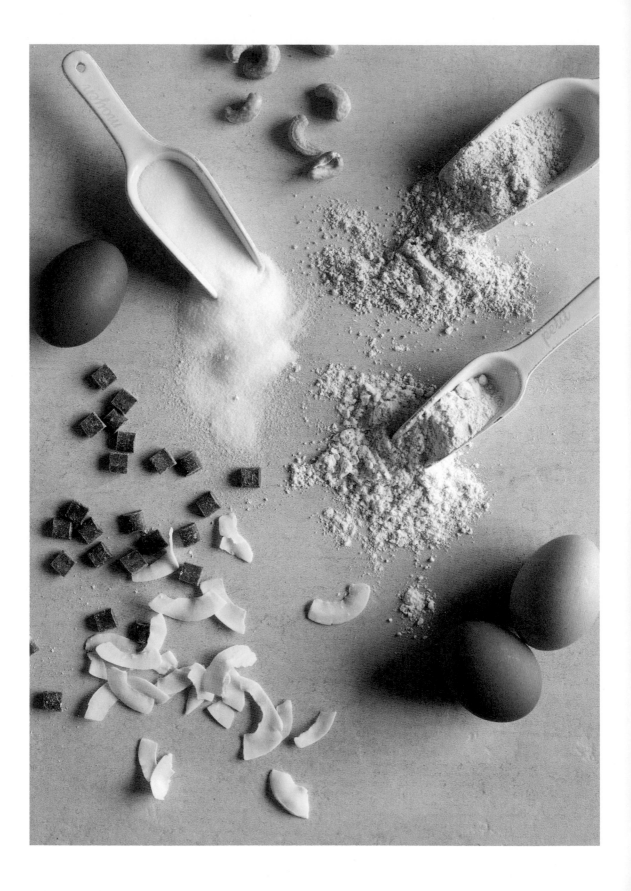

Introduction

I'm so excited about this book. It's the perfect follow-on from my previous three books in the Flexible series, *The Flexible Vegetarian, The Flexible Pescatarian* and *The Flexible Family Cookbook*, all of which offer a varied selection of recipes to suit differing wants and needs. All recipes come with suggested ingredient swaps and alterations throughout, giving the recipes unique flexibility to keep everyone happy.

What I came to realise after the *Flexible Family Cookbook* was released, is that baking is an area that can be really challenging for many people, particularly when it comes to cooking for individual dietary requirements. More often than not, when it comes to baking we're cooking for more than just ourselves, so having a cookbook with recipes that can be suitable for numerous requirements and occasions, is a handy book to have indeed.

I've always loved baking: when I was a little girl, I couldn't wait to get stuck into making biscuits and cakes with both my grandmothers and my mum. They were very patient and I'm sure we had many disasters along the way! However, their enthusiasm made it all the more enjoyable – as well as licking the mixing spoons, and tucking into the delicious results as quickly as possible.

It's the process of baking that I enjoy, from the preparation – measuring, mixing, blending – through to the cooking and waiting for the end result to come out, smelling amazing and looking beautifully baked. Then there's the finishing touches, with assembling and decoration.

I think for many of us it's the feeling of nostalgia that makes us love baking so much. Many children start off learning how to cook by baking biscuits, cookies or cupcakes. The aroma in the kitchen when baking is impossible to forget. For many, baking can be a form of relaxation, a way in which to switch off from the outside world. For others, it's the indulgence of tucking into a home-baked treat.

There's definitely a science behind baking that has to be taken into consideration. To create a perfect bake you need the correct balance of ingredients. Simply throwing a handful of this or that won't work in many baking recipes, so before you get into making these recipes, I suggest you have a set of scales, measuring spoons and measuring cups or jugs handy for the best possible results.

When it came to putting the recipes together for each chapter, I desperately wanted to make sure I was accommodating as many dietary requirements as possible without compromising flavour or appeal, and I hope you'll agree that the recipes in each chapter do offer plenty for everyone. The book is set out into six chapters, with a not-to-be missed dietary index at the end.

Savoury

To kick things off, I'm starting with a chapter of savoury bakes. Here you'll find delicious savoury scones, tempting tarts, irresistible sausage rolls, protein-packed muffins, comforting pasties and spiced patties. Vegetarian, vegan and pescatarians are all thought about within these recipes as well as other dietary requirements.

Breads

There is something deeply satisfying about making your own bread, and in this chapter there are so many different types to choose from: gluten-free, shaped breads, breakfast offerings, basic, quick, rich, wholesome and rustic breads. There's even a 'sourdough' recipe…I had to get onto the trend somehow, though my version is not quite as you'd expect.

Cakes and traybakes

In this chapter you'll find a variety of cakes and bakes for every occasion, and to enjoy at any time throughout the day using different flavours, textures and techniques. There are individual cupcakes, celebration cakes, everyday cakes, seasonal fruity cakes, indulgent traybakes, portable bakes, all of which are utterly delicious, offering something for everyone.

Biscuits and cookies

Such fun to make and often ready to eat in no time at all, biscuits and cookies have the added benefit of having a longer shelf life than other baked goodies. Here you'll find classic biscuits with a twist, delicate melt in-the-mouth biscuits, sandwich biscuits and there's even a very large cookie to share (or keep to yourself should you wish!).

Pastries

There is a lovely selection of recipes in this chapter, using numerous types of pastry, from ready-made puff pastry, choux pastry, shortcrust, pastry using different types of flour and even a chocolate pastry.

Puddings and desserts

From indulgent to light and refreshing, here you can find a recipe to finish off your meal perfectly, whether it's for a dinner party, Sunday lunch, celebration meal or your simple weekday dinner.

Dietary index

This dietary index is a valuable time-saving reference guide. Those indexed are: dairy-free, gluten-free, nut-free and sesame-free, egg-free and vegan.

I hope you'll find plenty of recipes in this book, with suitable flexibility that works for you as well as your family and friends' requirements. This time round trying out these recipes was slightly different as I was writing this book during lockdown due to the COVID pandemic. It was a challenge I embraced so rather than sharing my bakes in person, I found myself posting goodies to family members I couldn't see and leaving parcels on my neighbours' doorsteps. This turned out to be a great way of cooking for people with varying dietary requirements that I may not have connected with if it hadn't been for the unusual situation we found ourselves living in. They were extremely grateful and gave me some fantastic feedback that I worked into the recipes.

Please do enjoy these bakes and let their flexibility work for you.

Happy flexible baking! Jo x

The flexible baker's store cupboard

When it comes to flexible baking there are a selection of core ingredients that feature quite a lot in this book. It's worth keeping your kitchen well stocked, so you're always at the ready to tackle some flexible baking any time the requirement arises.

Flour

The base to the majority of these baking recipes uses flour in some form.

Plain flour and self-raising flour – the most commonly used wheat flours. You can make your own self-raising flour by mixing 3 teaspoons baking powder with 250g/9 oz/1¾ cups plain flour.

Strong bread flour – this has a higher protein content and therefore more gluten than a standard plain flour, so it's ideal for making springy textured bread.

Rye flour – used to make bread, it's also great for pastry, offering a rich, dark, slightly fruity flavour. Even though rye is a grass it still contains some gluten.

Spelt flour – great to use as an alternative to plain flour for added texture and flavour and for anyone requiring a lower gluten content in their baking (it still contains some gluten).

Gluten-free and flour alternatives

For gluten-free baking, there are some fantastic gluten-free flour blends available to buy that can commonly be used as a direct swap when a recipe calls for plain or self-raising flour. I have suggested using it as a flexible option in many recipes in this book. However, you'll see that I like to use other alternatives as well.

Gram (chickpea) flour – this is made from ground chickpeas so there is a pretty distinctive flavour to this flour, but used in the correct recipes it's absolutely delicious and very versatile.

Buckwheat flour – a nutritious wholegrain flour, with a distinctive, robust, earthy taste. It is in fact a herb, related to rhubarb and sorrel. Great to use in breads and pastries.

Coconut flour – high in fibre with a delicious distinctive flavour. Be wary about doing a straight swap for a wheat flour in a recipe, as it tends to absorb a lot more liquid creating a drier bake.

Cornflour – great to use as a thickening agent in baking.

Oats – I use these a lot as an alternative to plain flour in my recipes. Simple porridge oats (gluten-free) can be blended in a food processor to a fine powder.

Polenta – also known as fine cornmeal, it is a naturally gluten-free ingredient and wonderful in baking.

Nuts and seeds – many of the recipes in this book use nuts, almonds, hazelnuts, walnuts, cashew, pistachio nuts etc. When ground they're a wonderful gluten-free alternative to using flour and also add moisture due to their higher oil content. Ground almonds are easy to get hold of, however, any nut can be ground in a food processor until finely ground. If making a large batch, it's best stored and used directly from the freezer to keep fresh. Ground seeds are a superb nut-free alternative. Pumpkin, pine nut (yes, they are a seed!) or sunflower seeds can all be finely ground and used as ground nuts would be.

Dairy and alternatives

Milk – there is a wide range of dairy-free or plant-based milks available, both long life or fresh, that can all be used in exactly the same way as dairy milk in baking. Try and use an unsweetened variety if possible. Some of the recipes in this book specify which one to use as their flavour will fit better, however, on the whole I suggest using whichever you prefer: soya, nut milks (almond, hazelnut, cashew etc.), coconut, oat or rice milk.

Butter – unless the recipe states otherwise, I use unsalted butter in baking – that way the exact amount of salt can be controlled for specific recipes. Vegan, dairy-free or plant-based butter alternatives such as margarine can be used in most cases. I recommend you check they contain a minimum of 80 per cent fat and avoid using spreads, since they contain too much water. Coconut oil is another fantastic alternative to dairy butter. It can have a strong aroma and flavour, so unless you specifically want a coconut taste, it's better to use a refined one specifically for cooking.

Buttermilk – a common ingredient used in baking, though not always easy to get your hands on. A great substitute is a low-fat plain natural yoghurt, or you can make your own buttermilk by mixing 250ml/9 fl oz/ 1 cup milk (dairy or plant-based) with 1 tablespoon lemon juice or vinegar. Leave for 5–10 minutes to thicken and appear to curdle.

Eggs and alternatives

In baking, eggs act both as a raising agent and as a binder of ingredients. All of the recipes in this book use UK size large eggs, ideally free-range or organic. Often people think eggs are a dairy product, but they're not. For anyone with an egg allergy or intolerance, or those following a vegan diet, there are some fantastic alternatives that work for most recipes. Here's a few ideas you can use. Each of these = 1 egg.

Aquafaba – use 3 tablespoons, whisked until frothy – brilliant for binding and also making a vegan meringue. Aquafaba is simply the drained water from a can of chickpeas. Make sure to keep the chickpeas for a future meal.

Chia seeds or ground flaxseeds – use 1 tablespoon chia seeds or ground flaxseeds mixed with 3 tablespoons cold water and leave for 10 minutes to thicken and become gloopy like egg white.

Egg replacement powder – I haven't use it in any of these recipes, but it can be a useful ingredient to have if you are cooking egg-free recipes all the time.

Fruit or vegetable purée – 40–50g /1½–2oz puréed cooked apple, pear, pumpkin or ripe banana can help bind loaf cakes or muffins. Also wonderful in pancake batters. Choose according to your recipe as the flavour will be apparent in the end result.

As egg is often used as a raising agent in baking, you'll see many of the recipes use a combination of bicarbonate of soda and vinegar (or lemon juice), which react forming carbon dioxide, a powerful raising agent. As you go through the chapters, you'll see my preferred egg alternative suggestions in the Flexible sections.

Sugar and sweeteners

I've used various sugars in this book but the main ones are:

Caster sugar – the most commonly used sugar in many baking recipes. Its fine granules dissolve quickly. You can use golden or white.

Icing sugar – this powdery sugar dissolves upon hitting moisture and is essential for making frosting, icing and decorations. If you run out, then you can blend caster or granulated sugar in a food processor until it's fine and powdery and then use in the same way as icing sugar.

Soft light brown sugar – this has a delicious caramel flavour and often gives a slightly softer end result, particularly when used in biscuits or cookies.

Other sugars that occasionally appear in the following recipes are:

Demerara sugar – with larger toffee-coloured crystals that add crunch and texture to the top of crumbles, streusels and cookies

Muscovado sugar – this naturally contains molasses and gives a darker colour, moist texture and deep flavour to baking.

Golden syrup, maple syrup and honey feature quite a lot in these recipes. Do keep in mind that honey isn't suitable for a vegan diet, but both maple and agave syrup are a perfect swap.

Oil

Sunflower oil – the more versatile of oils to use in baking as it has a neutral flavour. It's suitable for vegans, vegetarians and those following gluten-free and dairy-free diets. It works well in many cake recipes and those made using melted butter. As it is liquid at room temperature, it helps keep the cake moist for longer.

Olive oil – for sweet baking recipes, opt for a light olive oil to avoid any strong flavour affecting the end result. Save the extra virgin olive oil for the savoury recipes.

Bicarbonate of soda and baking powder

Both essential in baking for giving rise and lift. If required, make sure you check the packaging for gluten-free versions.

Yeast

For ease and convenience, I like to use dried yeast. All recipes in this book use fast-action dried yeast. It's a granulated style yeast and comes in 7g/2¼ teaspoon sachets and can be added straight to dried ingredients. Don't confuse this with active dry yeast, which has to be 'bloomed' in warm water before using.

Vanilla

A very versatile natural flavour taken from the root of the vanilla orchid plant. It comes in many forms: liquid (extract), the whole pod that is split and seeds scraped out, powder and my favourite to use in baking, vanilla bean paste. For best flavour, be sure to use the real thing and avoid using vanilla flavouring.

Spices

A variety of spices are always useful to have on hand for all cooking, though the two spices I use most in baking are ground cinnamon and ground ginger. Both of which add a warmth and subtle flavour when used in small quantities, or really pack a punch when increased.

Chocolate and cocoa

I like to use dark chocolate with a 70 per cent cocoa solid as it has good balance of strength and flavour. If required, dairy-free or vegan dark, milk or white chocolate can be used as an alternative.

Cocoa powder is dairy-free and gluten-free (although do check the packaging), and an ideal ingredient to have in your cupboard all the time.

Where possible, choose a cocoa powder that uses the Dutch process, which is richer in flavour and deeper in colour.

Vinegar

Apple cider vinegar or white wine vinegar both react with bicarbonate of soda as a powerful raising agent, which is particularly useful when doing any egg-free or vegan baking.

Xanthan gum

This is a really useful addition to many gluten-free baking recipes, as it gives a stronger crumb texture and reduces crumbling.

Salt

I use two types of salt: **fine sea salt** when I want it to evenly distribute and flavour the entire bake: and **flaked sea salt** to give added crunch or a pop of salty flavour within a recipe or to sprinkle on top before or after baking for crunch and bite.

Dietary icons

Included in each recipe are icons to help you choose a recipe at a glance:

VEGAN

NUT/SESAME-FREE

DAIRY-FREE

EGG-FREE

GLUTEN-FREE

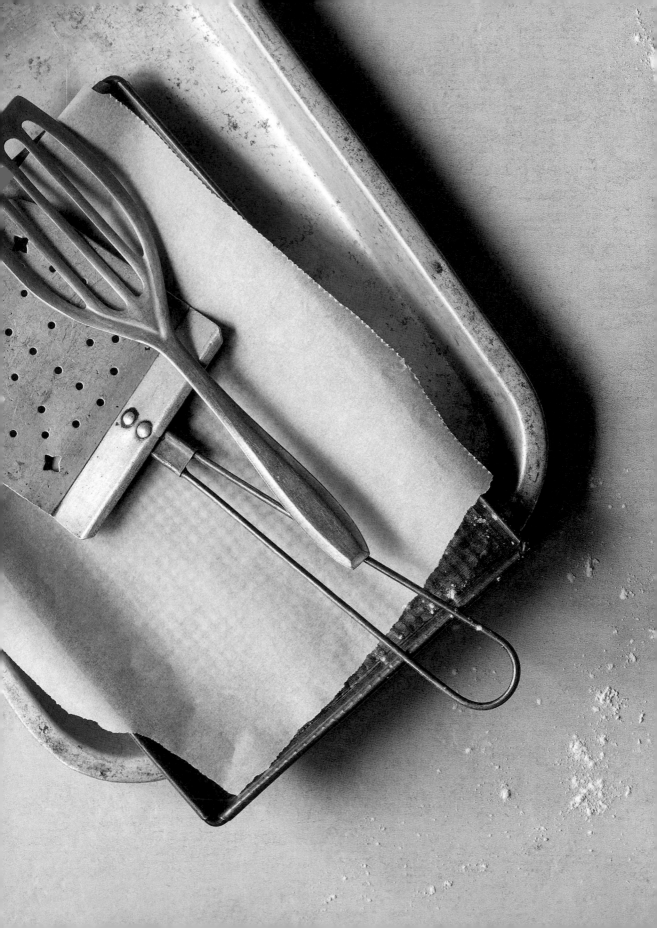

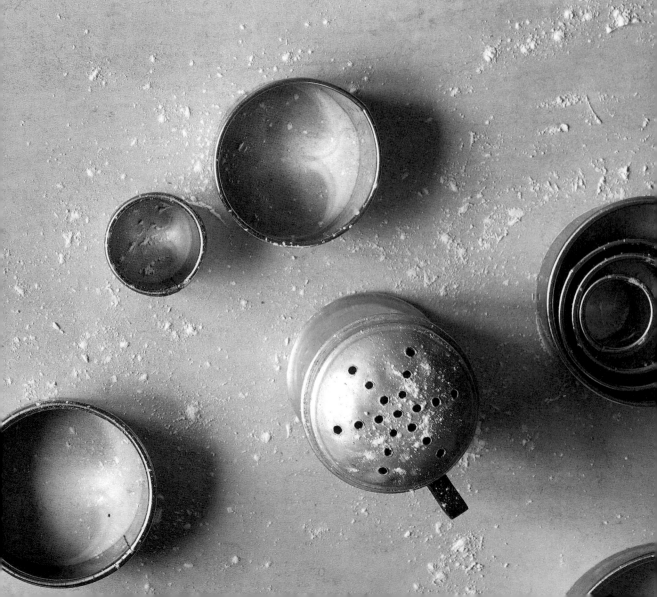

savoury

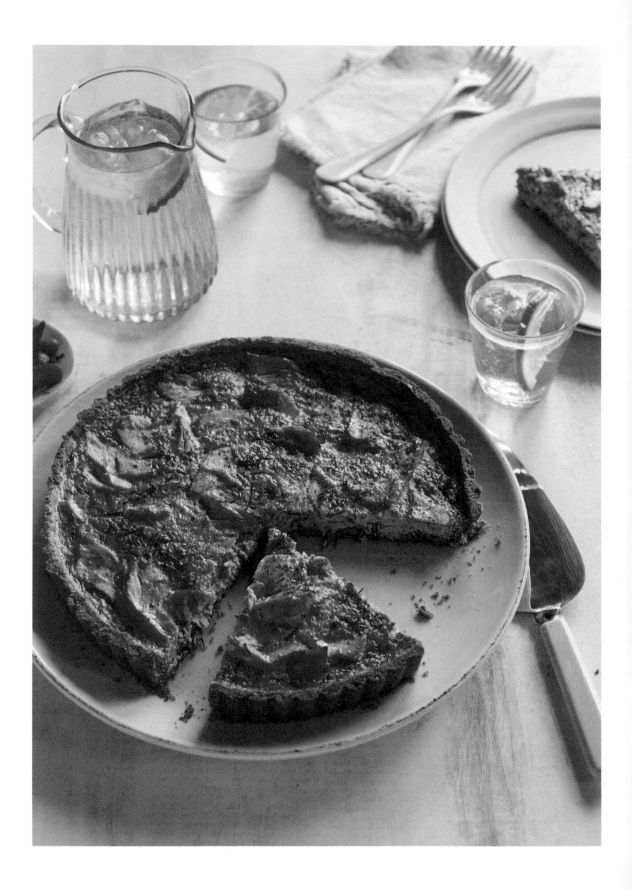

Salmon, dill and rye tart

*I've given a classic quiche a
Scandinavian twist with a rich
wholesome rye pastry, fresh salmon
and plenty of aromatic dill. It's packed
with flavour and a wonderful go-to tart
for supper, lunch or part of a sharing
platter with salads and charcuterie.
A mix of pickled gherkins, sliced
beetroot, avocado, red onion and
soured cream is a favourite side salad
of mine to serve alongside this tart.*

*This makes one large tart, although
you can easily make this into
individual ones if you wish.*

For the pastry

175g/6 oz/1⅓ cups rye flour, plus extra
   for dusting

½ tsp baking powder

½ tsp flaked sea salt

65g/2½ oz/¼ cup butter, chilled and diced,
   plus extra for greasing

65g/2½ oz/¼ cup cream cheese

2 tbsp milk

For the filling

300g/10½ oz skinless salmon fillet

olive oil

4 eggs

200g/7 oz/1 cup soured cream

25g/1 oz dill, roughly chopped

flaked sea salt and freshly ground
   black pepper

Prep 25 minutes / **Cooking** 45 minutes / **Serves** 6

To make the pastry, put the flour, baking powder and salt into a
large bowl or food processor. Add the butter and rub or blitz to a
fine crumb. Add the cream cheese and half of the milk, and bring
everything together until you have a dough, adding the remaining
milk if required. You should end up with a soft dough consistency.

Grease a 24cm/9 inch tart tin or pie dish with butter ready for the
pastry. Knead the dough lightly on a floured surface then roll out
thinly, turning a quarter turn every time you roll. Transfer to the
greased tin, pressing the pastry into the edges. Patch up any cracks
or breaks with pastry. Trim the edges and place in the fridge for
about 1 hour to chill. Keep any pastry trimmings back should they
be required to patch up any pastry cracks once baked.

Heat the oven to 200°C/180°C fan/400°F/gas 6. Line the pastry
case with baking parchment and pour in some baking beans,
uncooked rice or dried beans. Sit on a baking tray and bake for
15 minutes, then remove the parchment and beans and bake for
a further 8 minutes until the pastry is just turning golden.

While the pastry case is cooking, you can bake the salmon. Sit the
salmon fillets on a piece of foil and season with salt. Drizzle with
oil and loosely wrap to seal into a parcel. Pop in the oven while the
pastry case bakes and cook for the final 8 minutes.

Beat the eggs and soured cream together and season. Stir in the
dill and pour into the pastry case. Flake the salmon into the filling
and carefully transfer to the oven. Bake for 20–25 minutes until the
filling is just set and turning golden. Serve warm or cold.

Flexible

Gluten-free: *rye flour is extremely low in gluten, but if it's a completely
gluten-free pastry you require, you can use buckwheat flour, which has
an equally delicious nuttiness that rye flour provides.*

Vegetarian: *a fabulous swap for salmon in this tart is aged feta cheese
which has a deeper flavour and works really well with the aromatic dill
and nutty pastry. Coarsely crumble 300g / 10½ oz feta cheese into the
tart case before adding the egg and dill mixture. Bake as above.*

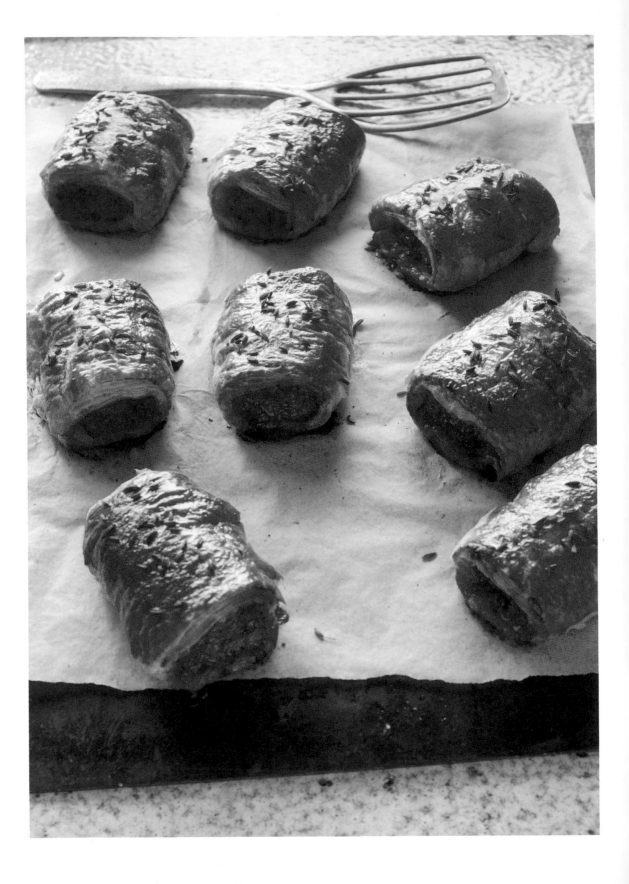

Chicken and chorizo sausage rolls

Oh wow – I have to say these are utterly delicious and really easy to make. I've even won my son Olly over with this recipe, who claims not to like sausage rolls. He'll ask for these most weekends. Luckily, they freeze really well, so when I make a batch, I'll freeze a few before they go in the oven, baking from frozen and adding on an additional 10 minutes of cooking time.

---

1 tbsp olive oil

1 red onion, finely chopped

½ red chilli, finely chopped

2 tsp fennel seeds

2 garlic cloves, crushed or grated

1 tbsp sherry vinegar or red wine vinegar

200g/7 oz chicken mince

175g/6 oz cooking chorizo sausages, skins removed and discarded

2 tbsp parsley, chopped

320g/11 oz sheet ready rolled puff pastry

1 egg, beaten, for glazing

flaked sea salt and freshly ground black pepper

Prep 30 minutes / **Cooking** 30 minutes / **Makes** 8

Heat the oil in a saucepan and add the onion, chilli and half of the fennel seeds. Cook for about 5 minutes until the onion has softened. Add the garlic and vinegar and cook for a further minute or until the liquid has cooked away. Remove from the pan and put in a large mixing bowl to cool.

Add the chicken mince, chorizo sausage meat and parsley to the bowl. Season with salt and pepper and mix well. It is best to do this by hand, so everything is evenly mixed. Or you can briefly mix in a food processor but don't overmix as it will become pasty.

Heat the oven to 200°C/180°C fan/400°F/gas 6. Line a baking tray with baking parchment.

Unroll the pastry and cut into two long strips. Divide the sausage filling between the centre of both strips and brush the beaten egg along one long side of each. Roll the other side of pastry over the filling and press down to seal. Using a sharp knife, cut each roll into 4, giving you 8 sausage rolls in total.

Put the sausage rolls on the baking tray, sealed side down and brush with beaten egg. Sprinkle over the reserved fennel seeds and bake for 25–30 minutes until golden and crisp. Serve warm or cold.

Flexible

Gluten-free: make sure the chorizo sausages are gluten-free and use a gluten-free puff pastry.

Vegan: for the filling, sauté 1 onion and ½ teaspoon dried chilli flakes in 1 tablespoon olive oil until soft. Increase the heat and add 250g/9 oz finely chopped portobello mushrooms. Cook until the mushrooms are soft and all the excess water has cooked away. Mix in 200g/7 oz finely crumbled firm tofu, 2 tablespoons dark miso paste, 1 tablespoon tomato purée, 2 teaspoons rice vinegar and 1 tablespoon chopped chives. Season with ½ teaspoon salt. Cook for a few minutes until the excess water has cooked out. Leave to cool. Assemble the sausage rolls as above, making sure you use a vegan puff pastry (most are unless labelled 'all-butter'). Brush the top with olive oil and scatter with sesame seeds or chopped peanuts and bake.

Sweet onion and blue cheese swirls

Not quite a bread or a pastry, these light and fluffy cheesy twirls are very hard to resist. I like to serve them with a bowl of soup or a tomato-based stew, but they'd be just as good served with some salad or on their own as a snack or sharing starter. If blue cheese isn't your thing, then have a play around with other soft cheeses. These are best eaten the day that they are made.

---

2 tbsp olive oil

1 large onion, finely sliced

1 tbsp balsamic vinegar

1 tbsp caster (superfine) sugar

325g/11½ oz/2½ cups self-raising (self-rising) flour, plus extra for dusting

250ml/9 fl oz/1 cup buttermilk or natural yoghurt

2 tbsp olive oil, plus extra for drizzling

1 tbsp sage leaves, finely chopped

1 tsp flaked sea salt

100g/3½ oz creamy blue cheese such as Dolcelatte or Gorgonzola, cut into pieces

freshly ground black pepper

Prep 40 minutes / **Cooking** 20 minutes / **Makes** 8

Heat the oil in a saucepan over a low heat and add the onion. Cook gently for around 15 minutes until soft and starting to become golden. Add the balsamic vinegar, sugar and season with salt and pepper. Cook for a further couple of minutes before removing from the heat and leaving to cool.

Heat the oven to 200°C/180°C fan/400°F/gas 6. Line a baking tray with baking parchment.

Put the flour, buttermilk or yoghurt, oil, sage and salt in a large bowl. Using a round-ended knife, mix until you have a soft dough. Turn out onto a worktop dusted with flour and gently and briefly knead until you have a smooth dough.

Dust a rolling pin with flour, and making sure the worktop is also well floured, roll out the dough to a 20 x 30cm/8 x 12 inch rectangle and scatter over the caramelised onions and blue cheese. Roll up from the long side of the dough to create a long sausage shape. Using a sharp knife, cut into 8 even pieces. Sit, cut side up, on the baking tray in a ring shape so they are almost touching one another and drizzle the top with olive oil.

Bake for 20 minutes until golden brown and serve warm.

Flexible

Vegan: *use a plant-based yoghurt alternative and a vegan cheese of your choice, grated if it's a hard cheese.*

Flavour swap: *for a milder cheese, Brie or Camembert are a great alternative to the blue cheese. You can switch the herbs around in the dough; basil, chives or thyme are all very tasty. Thinly sliced roasted red (bell) peppers, chopped olives and sundried tomatoes can also be sprinkled onto the dough before rolling up.*

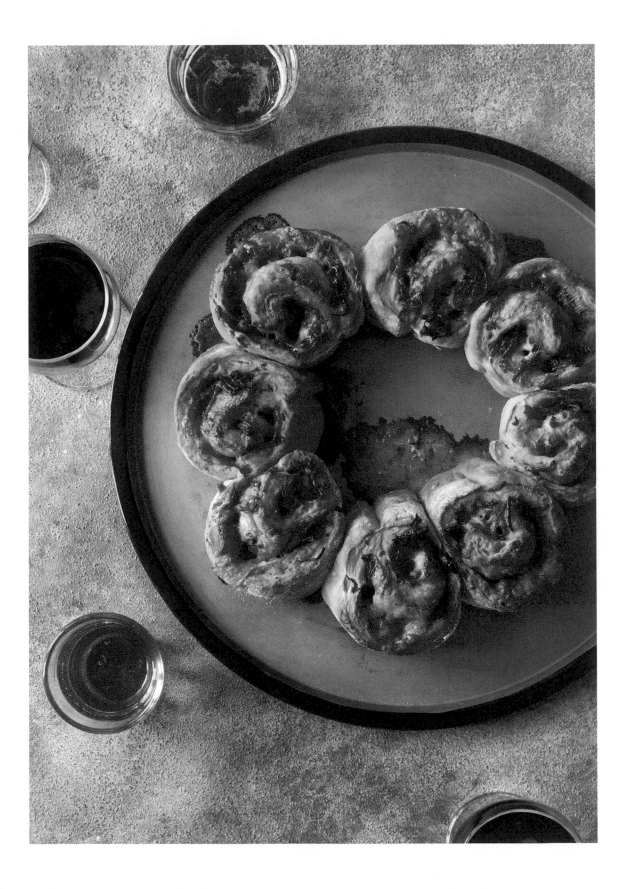

Cornish pasties

If you're going to go to the effort of making Cornish pasties, then it is well worth making them the 'proper' way. The rich flaky pastry is made using a combination of butter and lard with strong bread flour for extra pliability. The filling uses thinly sliced beef skirt (very tender with little fat), swede, potato, onion, butter and plenty of seasoning that all bake together within the pastry, creating a juicy gravy. Do take your time with the assembly and getting the classic crimped edge to the pasties so the end results not only taste utterly delicious but look impressive, too.

For the pastry

600g/1 lb 5 oz/4½ cups strong white
   bread flour, plus extra for dusting
150g/5½ oz/⅔ cup butter, chilled and
   diced
150g/5½ oz/⅔ cup lard, chilled and diced
1 tsp flaked sea salt
250ml/9 fl oz/1 cup ice-cold water
1 egg, beaten, for glazing

For the filling

400g/14 oz beef skirt steak,
   or stir-fry steak, finely chopped
1 medium onion, finely chopped
175g/6 oz potato, peeled and cut
   into small, slim pieces
175g/6 oz swede, peeled and cut
   into small, slim pieces
25g/1 oz butter, divided into 6
2 tsp flaked sea salt
1 tsp freshly ground
   black pepper

Prep 45 minutes / **Cooking** 45 minutes / **Makes** 6

To make the pastry, put the flour, butter, lard and salt in a large mixing bowl. Using your fingertips, lightly rub in the fats until you have a breadcrumb texture.

Gradually add the water, mixing with a knife to bring together, then use your hands to bring the pastry into a smooth ball, kneading briefly and lightly. Wrap in cling film and chill for around 1 hour.

Mix all of the filling ingredients together.

Heat the oven to 220°C/200°C fan/450°F/gas 8. Dust two baking trays with flour.

Divide the pastry into 6 and roll each one out on a floured surface into a circle, about 20cm/8 inch in diameter. Working on one pasty at a time, spoon one-sixth of the filling in the front half of the pastry circle, leaving a 1cm/½ inch border, and put a piece of butter on top.

Brush the edge with a little water, fold the pastry over the filling and seal. Starting on one side, place your thumb on top and index finger underneath, and with a firm movement, twist the pastry up towards you and down. Repeat to make a twisted rope effect along the edge, sealing the pasty. Sit on a baking tray and repeat with the other pasties.

Pierce a hole in the middle of each pasty and brush with beaten egg. Bake for 35 minutes, then turn off the oven and leave in the oven for 10 minutes to finish cooking. Remove from the oven and cool for 10 minutes before eating.

Flexible

Gluten-free: *The pastry has to be robust to hold the filling, so use a store-bought gluten-free puff pastry. It holds itself well during cooking and doesn't crack or crumble.*

Dairy-free: *use a firm, plant-based butter alternative or margarine and a vegetable lard to make the pastry.*

Vegetarian: *For a **sweet potato and chestnut** filling, mix together 350g / 12 oz finely sliced then roughly chopped sweet potato, 200g / 7 oz roughly chopped cooked chestnuts, a finely chopped red onion, a few chopped sage leaves and seasoning. Fill the pastry circles and top with 1 tablespoon crème fraîche, then seal and twist and bake as above.*

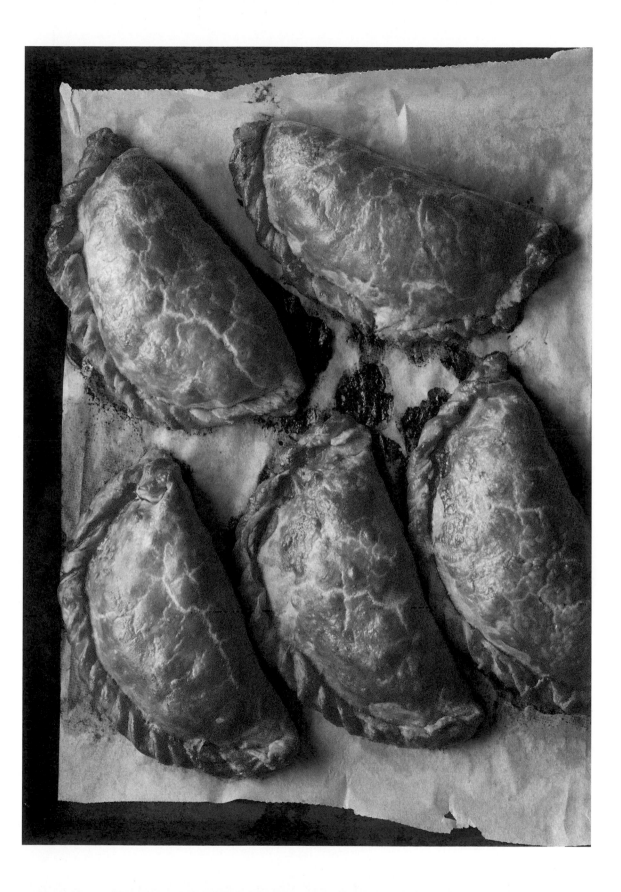

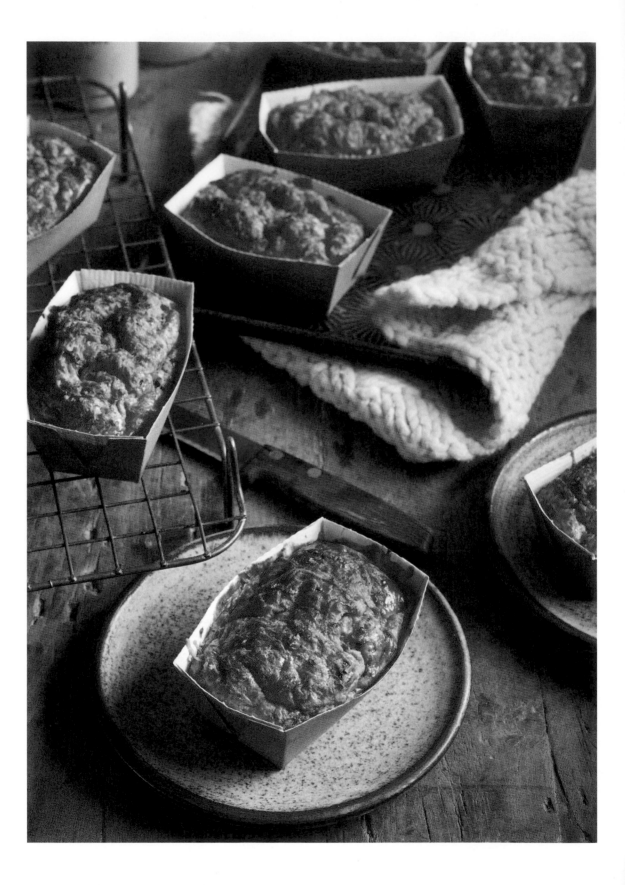

Ricotta, pumpkin and sage loaf muffins

These are incredibly easy to make – just looking at the length of the recipe gives that away! These super light muffins are packed with protein and contain very little flour in comparison to many savoury muffin recipes. They're a fantastic addition to a packed lunch or picnic as they transport well and can be served warm or cold. They also freeze well – simply defrost and eat cold or warm through when required. I like to make these in mini loaf cases but if you don't have any, then you can just line a muffin tin with 8–9 muffin cases instead.

300g/10½ oz peeled pumpkin or
   butternut squash, coarsely grated
250g/9 oz/generous 1 cup ricotta cheese
6 eggs, beaten
175g/6 oz/1⅓ cups self-raising
   (self-rising) flour
2 tbsp parsley, chopped
1 tbsp sage leaves, chopped
30g/1 oz Parmesan cheese, grated
20g/¾ oz pumpkin seeds
1 tsp flaked sea salt
freshly ground black pepper
olive oil, for drizzling

Prep 25 minutes / **Cooking** 25 minutes / **Makes** 8 mini loaves

Heat the oven to 200°C/180°C fan/400°F/gas 6. Place 8 mini loaf cases on a baking tray.

Put the grated pumpkin or butternut squash, ricotta, eggs, flour, parsley, sage, two-thirds of the Parmesan, the pumpkin seeds, salt and a good twist of black pepper in a large mixing bowl. Mix until combined, then divide between the loaf cases.

Scatter the remaining Parmesan over the top as well as a drizzle of olive oil. Bake for 25 minutes until the tops are lightly golden. Serve warm or cold.

Flexible

Gluten-free: *a gluten-free self-raising (self-rising) flour can be used instead of the self-raising wheat flour.*

Flavour swap: *to make **courgette and pesto muffins**, swap the pumpkin for 300g / 10½ oz grated courgette (zucchini). Place in a clean tea towel and squeeze out as much liquid as possible. Mix with 2 tablespoons pesto, 250g / 9 oz / generous 1 cup ricotta, 6 eggs (beaten), 175g / 6 oz / 1⅓ cups self-raising (self-rising) flour, 20g / ¾ oz Parmesan, 1 teaspoon flaked sea salt, freshly ground black pepper and 20g / ¾ oz pine nuts. Divide between 8–9 muffin cases and top with extra Parmesan and a drizzle of olive oil. Bake as above.*

Rustic tomato puttanesca tarts

This rich flaky pastry is very easy to make and a perfect base for individual tarts. You can make it with any topping you fancy (do have a go at the Flexible flavour swap suggestion below). Here, I'm sharing my all-time favourite. Sweet, caramelised onions with all of the classic flavours used in an Italian puttanesca sauce.

For the pastry

280g/10 oz/generous 2 cups plain (all-purpose) flour, plus extra for dusting

1 tsp flaked sea salt

175g/6 oz/¾ cup butter, chilled and diced

125–150ml/4–5 fl oz/½–⅔ cup ice-cold water

1 egg, beaten, for glazing

For the filling

2 tbsp olive oil, plus extra for drizzling

2 medium onions, finely sliced

1 tsp caster (superfine) sugar

4 anchovies in oil, finely chopped

½ tsp dried oregano

4–6 ripe, medium tomatoes, thinly sliced

16–20 pitted black olives, quartered

1 tbsp capers

½–1 red chilli, finely sliced

50g/2 oz finely grated Parmesan cheese

flaked sea salt and freshly ground black pepper

Prep 30 minutes, plus 30 minutes chilling / **Cooking** 30 minutes / **Makes** 4

To make the pastry, put the dry ingredients in a large bowl. Using your fingers, roughly rub in the butter, leaving larger chunks than if you were making a shortcrust pastry. This will make a flakier pastry. Drizzle over most of the water and bring everything together with your hands. Use the remaining water if required. Shape into a ball, wrap in cling film and put in the fridge to rest for 30 minutes.

To make the filling, heat the oil in a heavy-based frying pan over a low heat. Add the onions and sauté for 10 minutes until softened and starting to become lightly golden. Add the sugar, anchovies and oregano. Continue to cook for a further 5 minutes, stirring frequently. Remove from the heat and cool slightly.

Heat the oven to 200°C/180°C fan/400°F/gas 6. Line two baking trays with baking parchment and dust with flour.

Dust the worktop with flour. Remove the pastry from the fridge and divide into 4 balls. Roll out each ball about 3mm/⅛ inch thick, giving you circles of around 20cm/8 inch diameter. Spread the onions in the centre of the pastry circles, leaving a 2cm/¾ inch border. Arrange the tomato slices on top and scatter over the olives, capers and chilli, finishing with a good twist of pepper, a pinch of salt, scattering of Parmesan and a drizzle of olive oil.

Fold the rim of pastry up and over the edge of the tarts and brush the pastry with beaten egg. Bake the tarts for 25–30 minutes, until golden. Serve hot, warm or at room temperature.

Flexible

Vegan: use a plant-based butter alternative to make the pastry. Omit the anchovies and use ½ teaspoon flaked sea salt when cooking the onions for flavour. Use a vegan Parmesan-style cheese and brush the pastry with oil rather than egg.

*Flavour swap: to make **fig and prosciutto tarts**, omit the anchovies and divide the onions between the pastry circles. Arrange 3–4 sliced figs on top of the onions and add 4–6 slices of prosciutto torn into pieces. Scatter over a small handful of roughly chopped walnuts, season and drizzle with olive oil. Brush the pastry with egg and bake as above.*

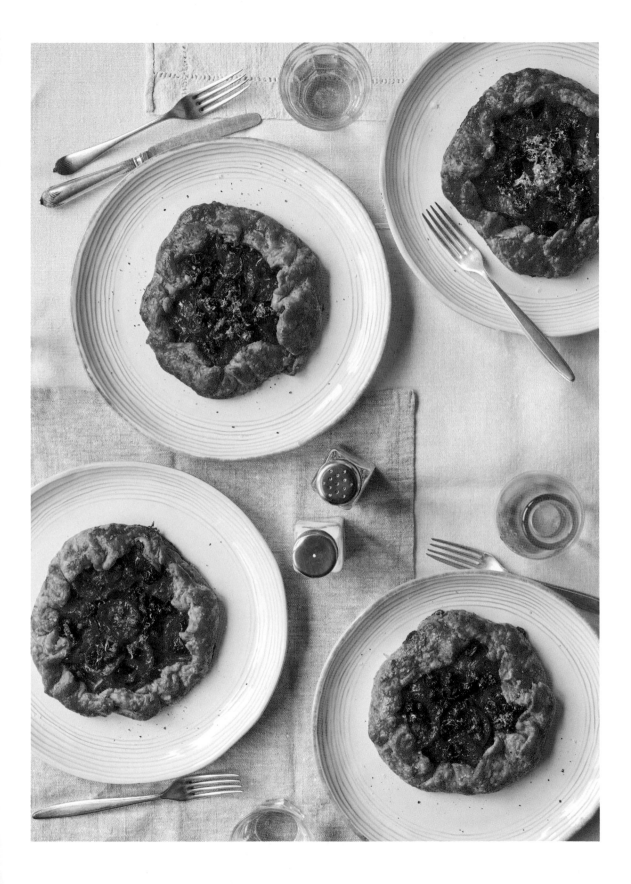

Spiced sweet potato strudel

If you're after a go-to vegan dish that's packed full of flavour and straightforward to make, then this is it. The Moroccan-inspired sweet potato and chickpea filling is encased in layers of flaky filo pastry, with each layer flavoured with lemon zest and aromatic herbs.

This versatile strudel can be served for all types of occasions; cut into small slices with salad for lunch, cold for a packed picnic or even as an impressive celebration centrepiece.

750g/1 lb 10 oz sweet potatoes, cut lengthways

40g/1½ oz/⅓ cup pine nuts

4–5 tbsp olive oil

1 large onion, finely sliced

1 tsp cumin seeds

½ tsp ground cinnamon

1–2 tsp harissa paste

400g/14 oz tin chickpeas (garbanzo beans), drained

75g/2¾ oz/½ cup sultanas (golden raisins)

1 tbsp mint leaves, chopped

1 tbsp parsley, chopped

1 tbsp coriander (cilantro), chopped

finely grated zest of 1 lemon

6 sheets filo pastry

flaked sea salt and freshly ground black pepper

2 tsp sesame seeds

Prep 40 minutes / **Cooking** 30–40 minutes / **Serves** 8–12

Heat the oven to 180°C/160°C fan/350°F/gas 4. Line a baking tray with baking parchment.

Place the sweet potatoes, cut side down, on the baking tray. Roast for 25–30 minutes until tender. Put the pine nuts on a small baking tray and lightly toast in the oven for 5 minutes. Set aside. Scoop the cooked potato flesh into a large bowl and mash with a fork.

Heat 2 tablespoons of the olive oil in a frying pan and cook the onion for 8 minutes until soft and turning golden. Add the cumin seeds and cinnamon and cook for a further minute or so. Spoon the onions into the sweet potatoes and add the harissa, chickpeas, sultanas, toasted pine nuts and season with salt and pepper.

In a separate bowl, mix together the chopped herbs and lemon zest.

Lay one sheet of filo pastry on top of a piece of baking parchment and brush the pastry generously with olive oil. Scatter with some of the lemony herbs and sit another piece of filo on top. Repeat until all of the filo sheets have been used. Spread the sweet potato filling over the filo, leaving a 2cm/¾ inch border all around the edge. Drizzle with oil and fold over the borders, holding in the filling.

Start rolling to create a log shape, finishing with the seam side down. Slide a baking sheet underneath the parchment. Brush the strudel with oil and scatter with the sesame seeds.

Bake for 30–40 minutes until the pastry is crisp and golden. Cool for about 20 minutes before slicing with a serrated knife.

Flexible

Nut-free: *if you want to avoid pine nuts, then leave them out and add a handful of chopped green olives in their place. To avoid sesame seeds, sprinkle the top with some nigella (black onion) seeds or leave plain.*

Gluten-free: *this filling works really well baked in a sheet of ready rolled gluten-free puff pastry. Make the filling as per the recipe and sit along the length of the pastry sheet. Fold over the short ends, then fold over the long sides creating a long sausage shape. Transfer to a baking tray, seam side down. Lightly slash the top a few times with a knife and brush with some olive oil. Scatter with the sesame seeds and bake as above.*

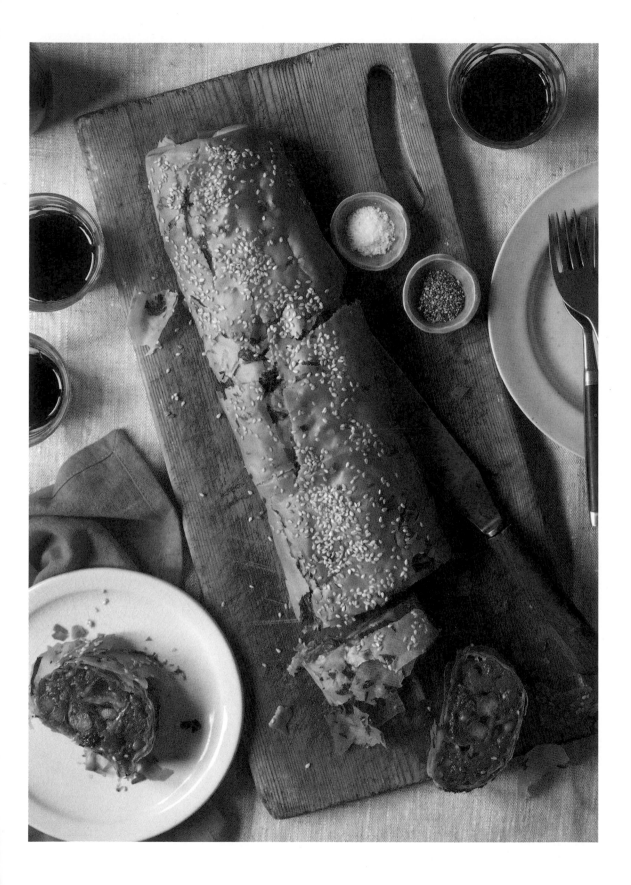

Smoky bacon scones

with salted maple butter

There is something very special about the combination of salty bacon and sweet maple syrup. They are often paired together with pancakes for breakfast, but here I've introduced them to light fluffy savoury scones.

Cut the dough into neat rounds with a pastry cutter or keep them more rustic and serve in wedges. Either way – serve warm, split in half and slathered with the salty maple butter.

For the scones

12 slices smoked streaky bacon,
   finely chopped

400g/14 oz/3 cups plain (all-purpose)
   flour, plus extra for dusting

1½ tsp baking powder

½ tsp bicarbonate of (baking) soda

½ tsp flaked sea salt, plus extra
   for sprinkling

175g/6 oz/¾ cup butter, chilled and diced

2 eggs

200ml/7 fl oz/generous ¾ cup buttermilk
   or natural yoghurt

For the maple butter

100g/3½ oz/½ cup butter

50ml/2 fl oz maple syrup

¼ tsp flaked sea salt

Prep 35 minutes / **Cooking** 15 minutes / **Makes** 8

Heat the oven to 200°C/180°C fan/400°F/gas 6. Line a large baking tray with baking parchment.

Put the bacon into a cold frying pan and put over a medium heat. Cook until the bacon is golden and crisp, cooking in its own fat. Drain on paper towel and cool the bacon in the fridge until completely cold.

Mix together the dry ingredients for the scones in a large bowl. Add the butter and lightly rub into the flour mix until you have a coarse crumb texture, lifting your hands as you rub to allow air into the flour. Stir the chilled bacon into the bowl, breaking up any clumps.

Beat one of the eggs into the buttermilk or yoghurt and pour into the bowl. Mix together quickly using a round-ended knife until just combined and turn out onto a floured worktop. Lightly fold together until you have a soft dough. Flatten into a rough circle about 2.5cm/ 1 inch thick. Rest for 5 minutes, then use a sharp knife to cut into 8 triangular wedges.

Transfer to the baking tray. Beat the other egg and brush the tops of the scones, sprinkle with salt and bake for 15 minutes until golden. These are best eaten warm on the day they are made. You can always freeze any before baking, for up to 1 month, and defrost at room temperature before baking when needed.

To make the butter, put all the ingredients in a bowl and beat really well until light and creamy, ideally using an electric mixer. Serve with the warm scones.

Flexible

Dairy-free: use a plant-based butter alternative such as baking margarine. Instead of the buttermilk or yoghurt, you can use 200ml / 7 fl oz / generous ¾ cup plant-based milk mixed with 1 tablespoon lemon juice. Stand for 5 minutes to allow to thicken and use as you would the buttermilk or yoghurt as above.

*Vegetarian: for **wholemeal Cheddar and chive scones**, swap 200g / 7 oz / 1½ cups plain (all-purpose) flour for 200g / 7 oz / 1½ cups plain (all-purpose) wholemeal (wholewheat) flour. Stir in 200g / 7 oz / 2 cups grated strong Cheddar cheese and 2 tablespoons chopped chives instead of the bacon. Sprinkle 75g / 2¾ oz / ⅓ cup grated Cheddar over the top of the glaze before baking. Serve with tomato chutney.*

Porcini, thyme and oat scones

Savoury scones are really delicious served alongside soups, stews, salads or if you need to eat on the go. I really wanted to include a savoury scone recipe that is suitable for both vegan and gluten-free diets. Unlike the more traditional scones, these are slightly denser in texture, due to the nature of the ingredients, and the flavour is rich and punchy. I love them served warm, cut in half and spread with a vegan cream cheese, red pepper paste or even some houmous.

15g/½ oz dried porcini mushrooms

4 tbsp freshly boiled water

175g/6 oz/1¼ cups oats (gluten-free), plus 1 tbsp

75g/2¾ oz/¾ cup ground almonds

2 tsp baking powder (gluten-free)

1 tsp bicarbonate of (baking) soda

2 tsp thyme leaves, roughly chopped, or 1 tsp dried thyme

½ tsp paprika

1 tsp flaked sea salt

125ml/4 fl oz/½ cup almond, oat or soya milk, plus extra for glazing

1 tbsp white wine vinegar or apple cider vinegar

100g/3½ oz/½ cup almond or cashew nut butter

2 tbsp sunflower or olive oil

Prep 30 minutes / **Cooking** 20 minutes / **Makes** 8

Heat the oven to 180°C/160°C fan/350°F/gas 4. Line a baking tray with baking parchment.

Put the dried mushrooms in a small bowl and pour over the hot water. Leave to absorb the liquid for 15 minutes.

Meanwhile, put the oats (keeping back the tablespoon of oats) in a food processor and blitz until you have a fine powder that resembles flour. Transfer to a large mixing bowl and mix in the ground almonds, baking powder, bicarbonate of soda, half of the thyme, the paprika and salt.

Strain the mushrooms (reserving any soaking liquid) and roughly chop. Add to the bowl of dry ingredients with the soaking liquid.

Add the milk, vinegar, nut butter and oil to a food processor and blitz briefly to mix together. Pour into the bowl and bring everything together to form a soft dough. Flatten with the palm of your hand and roll out with a rolling pin to 3cm/1¼ inch thick. Use a pastry cutter (I use one that's 5cm/2¼ inch in diameter) to cut out 8 scones, re-rolling any trimmings until all the dough is used up. Alternatively, you can shape the dough into a round disk and using a sharp knife, cut into 8 wedges. Sit on the baking tray, brush the top of the scones with a little milk and scatter over the remaining oats and thyme. Bake for 15 minutes until golden.

Leave to cool for a few minutes before serving warm. Best eaten on the day they are made.

Flexible

*Flavour swap: to transform these into **red pepper and walnut scones**, use 75g / 2¾ oz / ½ cup walnuts and blitz with the oats until fine. Use a hazelnut butter and milk, and use 100g / 3½ oz chopped roasted red (bell) pepper (from a jar) as an alternative to the mushrooms. Mix and bake as above.*

*For **Parmesan and sundried tomato scones** that are still gluten-free, omit the mushrooms and mix 60g/2 oz chopped sundried tomatoes and 60g/2 oz/¾ cup finely grated Parmesan cheese into the scone mixture. If the scone mixture seems too dry, just add a little extra milk to the dough until you have a soft pliable consistency. Bake as above.*

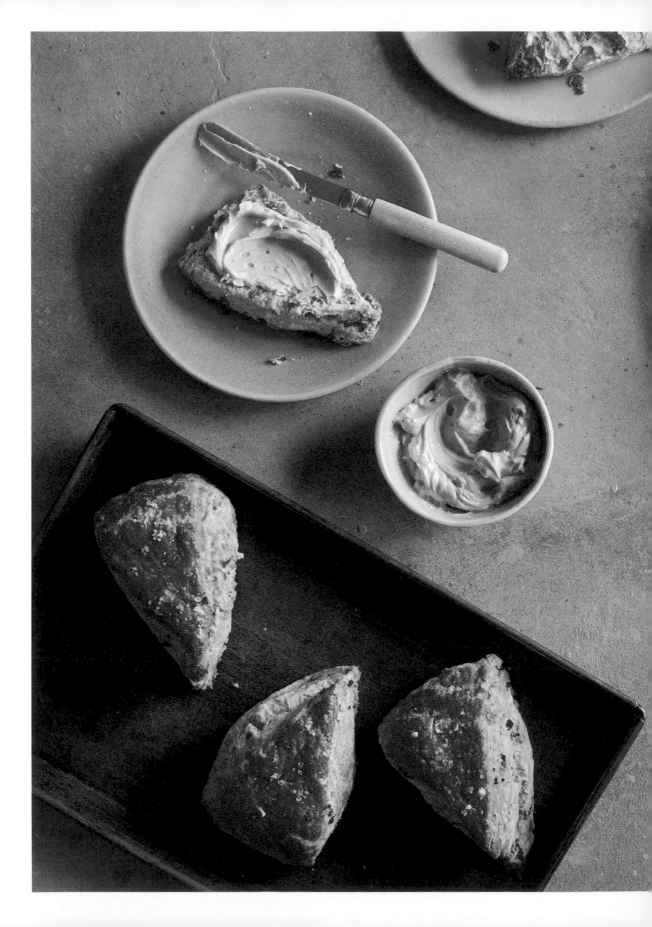

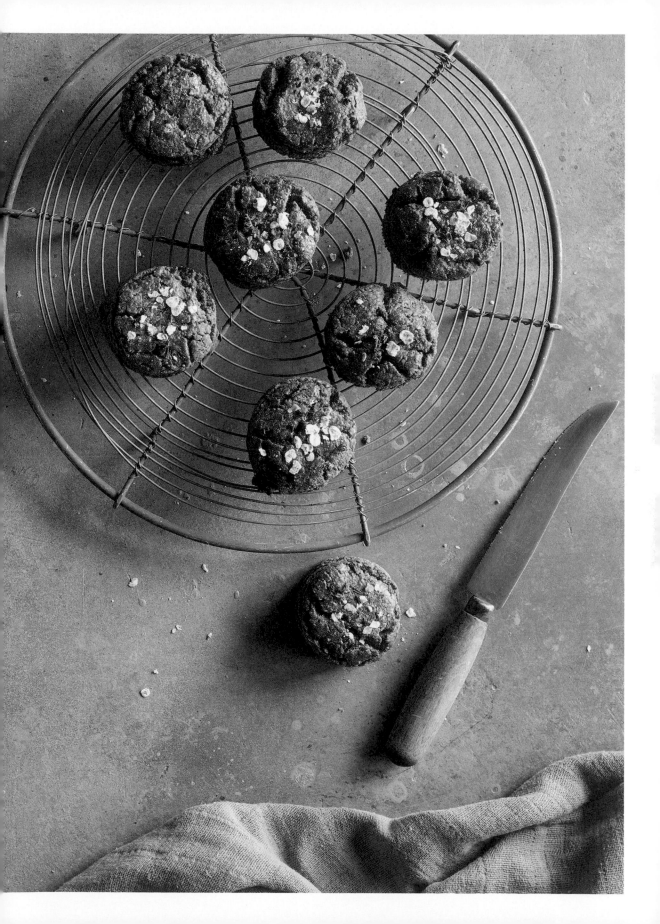

Golden vegetable patties

The idea for these colourful patties came from a recipe my children made in their cooking class at school although rather than making them using a standard wheat flour pastry like they did, I have made the these with gram (chickpea) flour. Not only does it have a great flavour that is ideal for savoury recipes, it's also naturally gluten-free. These little golden pockets are packed with veggies and ideal to make for lunch, picnics or for after school snacks.

For the pastry

300g/10½ oz/2¼ cups gram (chickpea) flour, plus extra for dusting

½ tsp xanthan gum

1 tsp ground turmeric

½ tsp fine sea salt

150g/5½ oz/⅔ cup butter, chilled and diced

1 egg, beaten, for glazing

For the filling

2 tbsp sunflower oil

1 small onion, finely diced

1 medium carrot, grated

1 small-medium sweet potato, peeled and grated

1 small-medium courgette (zucchini), grated

1 garlic clove, grated

1 tsp fresh root ginger, grated

½ red or green chilli, finely chopped

200g/7 oz tinned chopped tomatoes

flaked sea salt and freshly ground black pepper

Prep 30 minutes / **Cooking** 20 minutes / **Makes** 12

To make the pastry, put the flour, xanthan gum, turmeric and salt into a large bowl. Add the butter and rub the mixture together with the tips of your fingers until it looks like coarse breadcrumbs.

Add 150ml/5fl oz cold water and gently combine until you have a ball of soft slightly sticky dough, adding a little more water if required. The dough needs to be a little wet as this will absorb into the flour while resting. Cover in cling film and chill in the fridge while you make the filling.

Heat the oil in a frying pan and sauté the onion for 2 minutes until it starts to soften. Add the rest of the vegetables and aromatics. Cook for about 8 minutes until the vegetables are soft.

Stir in the tinned tomatoes and season. Cook for 5 minutes until thickened. Remove from the heat and let the filling cool.

Heat the oven to 180°C/160°C fan/350°F/gas 4.

Divide the pastry into 12 and roll into balls. Roll each one out into a circle, on a lightly floured worktop, to roughly 10cm/4 inches in diameter and about 5mm/¼ inch thick. Keep turning as you roll to prevent the pastry sticking to the worktop.

Place a spoon of your cooled filling in the middle of each pastry circle. Brush around the outside with beaten egg and fold each circle in half. Press the edges together to seal and use a fork to crimp them. Brush the surface with the egg and sit on a baking tray.

Bake for 20 minutes or until light golden brown. Allow to cool for 10 minutes before eating.

Flexible

Vegan: use a plant-based butter for the pastry. As an alternative for the egg, you can use water to seal the patties and brush the tops with olive oil.

Flavour swap: for **spiced lamb patties**, sauté 1 diced onion in 1 tablespoon sunflower oil until golden. Add 250g/9 oz lamb mince, 1 grated carrot, 2 grated garlic cloves, 1 teaspoon grated ginger and 1 tablespoon mild or medium curry powder. Fry over a high heat for 5 minutes until the meat is cooked through. Stir in 1 tablespoon tomato purée, season and leave to cool. Fill the patties and bake as above.

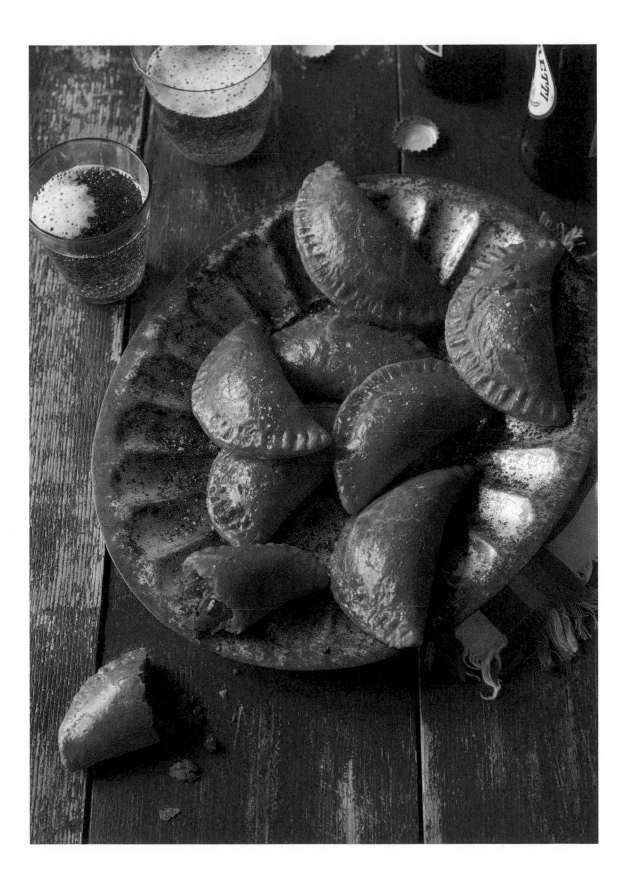

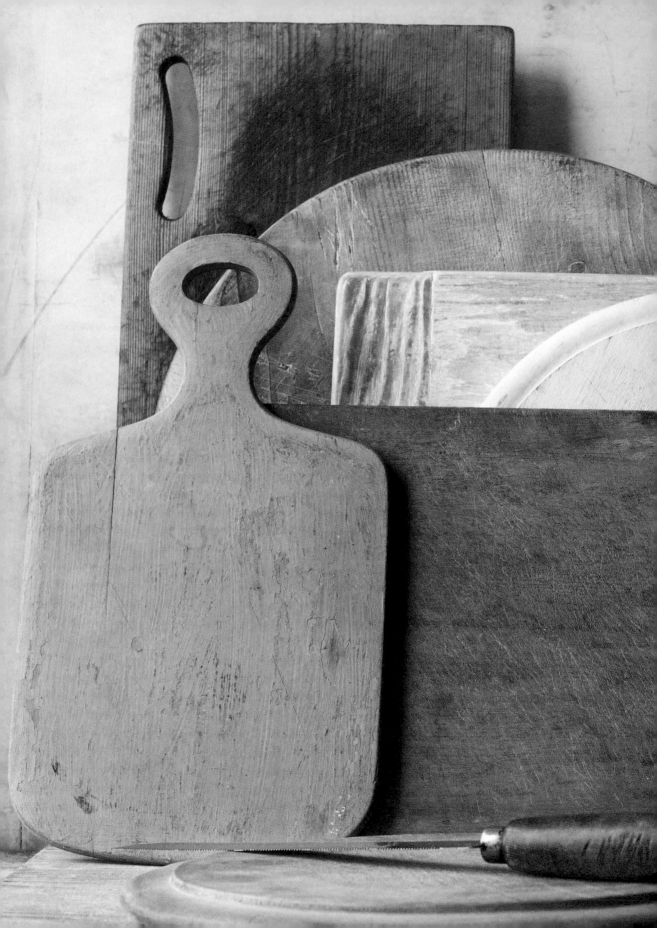

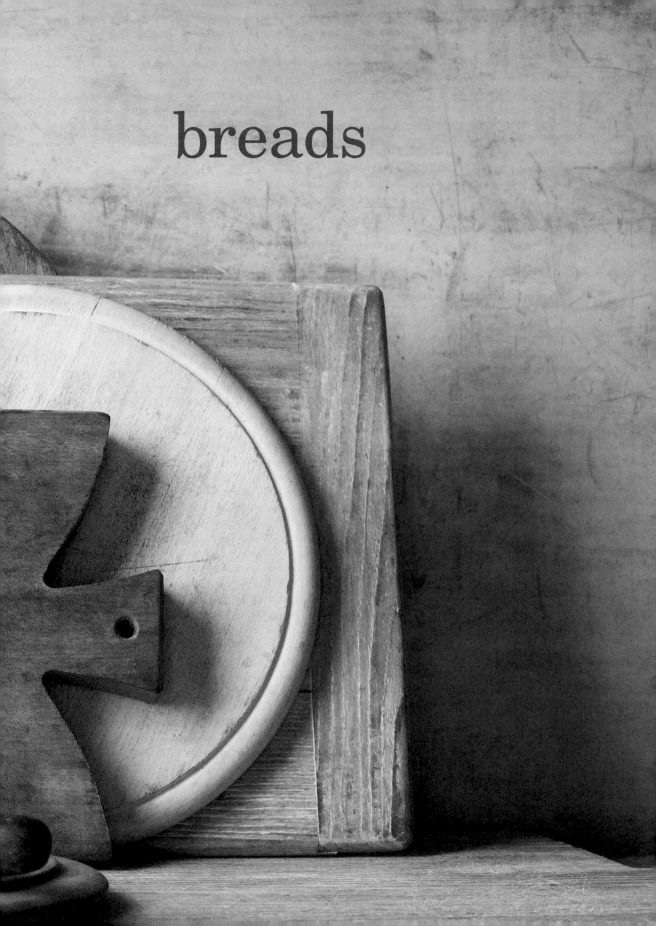

breads

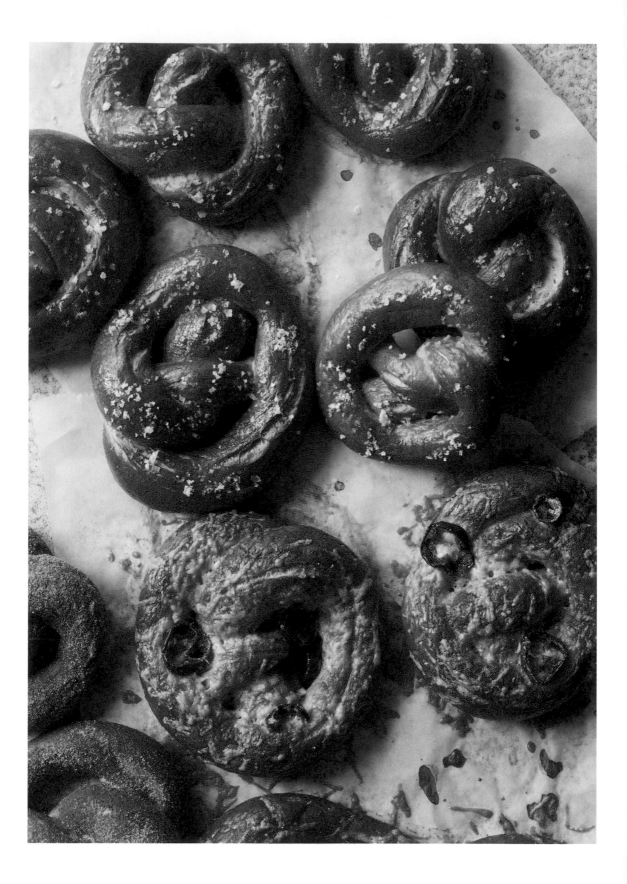

Soft pretzels

Homemade pretzels are surprisingly easy to make and give you the most amazing results. Make them once and I guarantee you'll make them again. You can bake them with a little flaked sea salt on top or mix things up a little and top them with Cheddar and spicy jalapeños, or an irresistible cinnamon-sugar coating. We all know our favourite in my house, so this really is a perfect recipe that will make everyone happy.

500g/1 lb 2oz/3¾ cups strong white bread flour, plus extra for dusting
7g/2¼ tsp fast-action dried yeast
25g/1 oz dark brown sugar
60g/2 oz/¼ cup butter, melted
1 tsp flaked sea salt, plus extra for sprinkling
1 tbsp bicarbonate of (baking) soda
1 egg, beaten, for glazing

Prep 55 minutes, plus 1 hour rising / **Cooking** 25 minutes / **Makes** 8

Put the flour, yeast and sugar in a large bowl, then stir to combine.

Measure 300ml/10 fl oz/1¼ cups lukewarm (around 40°C/100°F) water. Pour into the flour along with the melted butter and salt. Mix to form a dough, then turn out onto a floured surface to knead for about 10 minutes until smooth and elastic. Alternatively, do the whole process in an electric mixer using a dough hook.

Transfer the dough to a lightly oiled bowl. Cover with a damp tea towel or oiled cling film and leave in a warm place for about 1 hour, or until doubled in size.

Once risen, tip onto the worktop and divide into 8 pieces. Roll each piece into a long rope, about 60cm/24 inches long, trying not to knock out all of the air. Make a U-shape with each one, take the two ends and cross them over, then bring them down towards yourself and press into the base of the U-shape at 4 and 8 on a clock.

Heat the oven to 200°C/180°C fan/400°F/gas 6 and line two baking trays with baking parchment.

Fill a wide saucepan with about 1.8 litres/60 fl oz/7½ cups water and bring to a simmer. Add the bicarbonate of soda. One at a time, carefully immerse the pretzels into the water and cook for 20 seconds each side. Remove from the pan with a slotted spoon and sit on the baking tray. Repeat with the remaining pretzels.

Brush with beaten egg and sprinkle with sea salt. Bake for 20–25 minutes until deep, rich golden brown. Cool on a wire rack.

Flexible

Vegan: use a plant-based butter alternative or olive oil in the dough and rather than egg to glaze the pretzels you can brush with some olive oil before baking.

Flavour swap: to make **Cheddar and jalapeño pretzels,** top each pretzel with a handful of grated mature Cheddar cheese (you'll need about 175g/6 oz/2 cups for 8 pretzels) and 3–4 slices of pickled jalapeños and bake as above. Cover the top of the tray loosely with foil if the cheese starts to colour too much. Enjoy warm, dipped in a mix of equal parts honey and mustard.

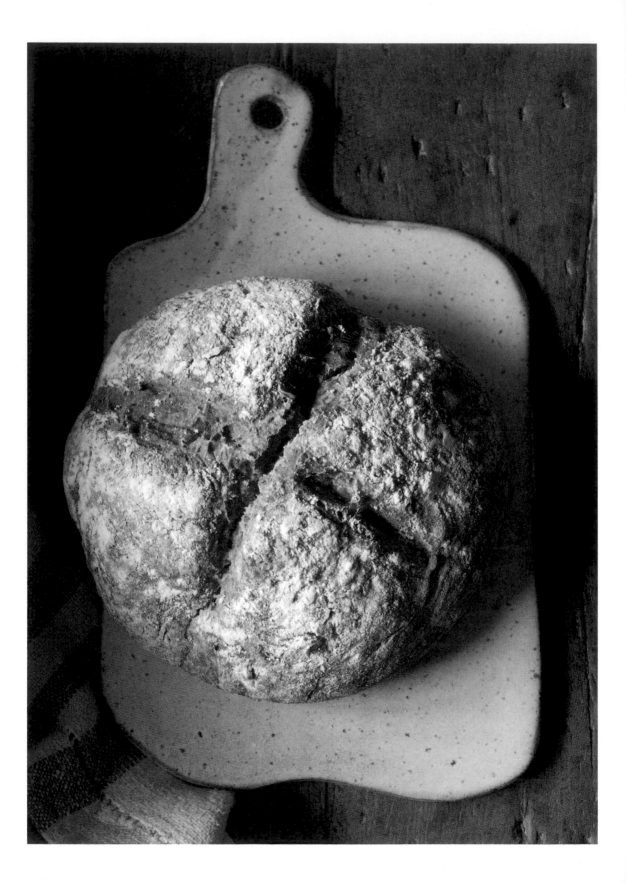

Quick soda bread

Making your own bread certainly need not be time consuming or hard work and this is a perfect example of just that, as soda bread doesn't require kneading or time to rise. Traditionally, it uses buttermilk to react with bicarbonate of soda to rise, however, buttermilk isn't always easy to get hold of, so this recipe uses some everyday ingredients – milk and vinegar – that work just as well. The end result is a soft, dense bread with the most incredible crust. Tear or cut into pieces and enjoy over a few days.

1½ tbsp white wine vinegar, apple cider
    vinegar or lemon juice
350ml/12 fl oz/1½ cups milk
225g/8 oz/1¾ cups plain (all-purpose)
    flour, plus extra for dusting
225g/8 oz/1¾ cups wholemeal flour
2 tsp soft brown sugar or caster
    (superfine) sugar
1 tsp bicarbonate of (baking) soda
½ tsp flaked sea salt, plus extra
    for sprinkling

Prep 15 minutes / **Cooking** 30 minutes / **Makes** 1 large loaf

Stir the vinegar or lemon juice into the milk and set aside for a few minutes for the milk to thicken and curdle slightly.

Heat the oven to 220°C/200°C fan/425°F/gas 7. Sprinkle some flour on a baking tray.

Put the flours, sugar, bicarbonate of soda and salt in a large bowl and stir well to combine. Make a well in the centre and pour in the milk mixture. Stir to form a sticky dough, then using floured hands bring the dough together to form a big ball. The dough should be soft but not too wet.

Sit the dough on the floured baking tray and cut a deep cross in the top of the dough with a knife, almost but not quite all the way through. Sprinkle over a little flour and some salt.

Bake in the oven for 30 minutes until it is golden and cooked through. To check, you can tap the base of the loaf and when cooked it will sound hollow.

Cool on a wire rack before slicing or tearing into chunks.

Flexible

Vegan: *switch the milk for a plant-based alternative. I really like to use oat milk for its mild flavour, but any will work and react in the same way when mixed with the vinegar or lemon juice.*

Flavour swap: *to make this loaf into a **cheese and onion soda bread**, stir 125g / 4½ oz / 1¾ cups grated mature Cheddar cheese and 1 teaspoon onion granules into the flour before adding the milk. Scatter the top with an additional 50g / 1¾ oz / ½ cup grated Cheddar and 1 teaspoon poppy seeds. If the cheese is becoming too golden before the loaf is ready, reduce the heat and cook for a little longer.*

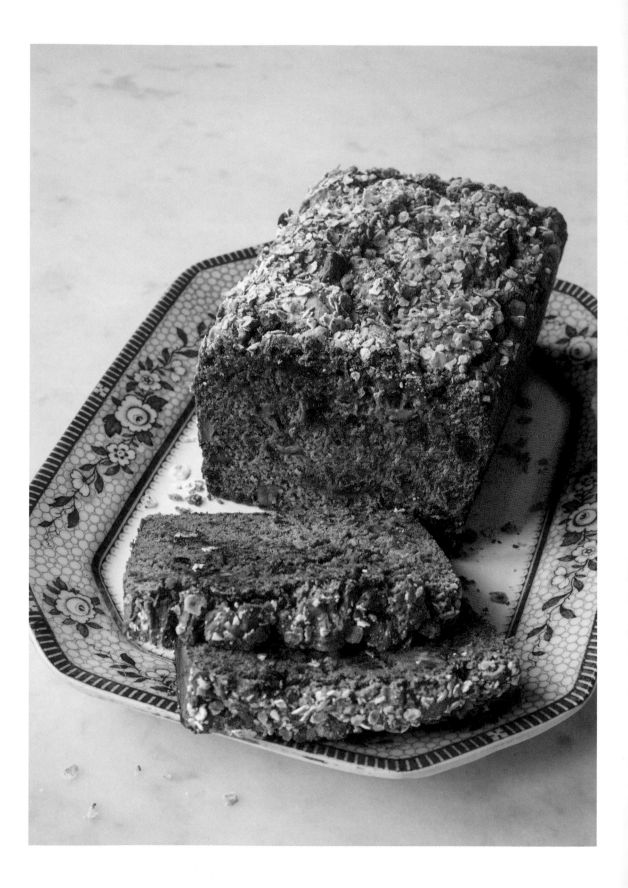

Breakfast muesli loaf

This loaf is packed with nutritious ingredients making it an ideal loaf to cut into for breakfast, keeping you full until lunchtime. It's gluten-free, which is a real bonus for those struggling to find suitable breakfast breads.

Serve sliced as it is, spread with butter and jam or honey, or it can also be toasted for a crunchier texture.

350g/12 oz/2⅔ cups buckwheat flour

1 tsp bicarbonate of (baking) soda

1 tsp ground cinnamon

½ tsp fine sea salt

2 eating apples, peeled and
   coarsely grated

75g/2¾ oz dried apricots, chopped
   into small pieces

75g/2¾ oz/¾ cup pecans, walnuts,
   cashews or hazelnuts, roughly chopped

40g/1¼ oz/¼ cup sunflower or pumpkin
   seeds

250ml/4 fl oz/1 cup apple or cranberry
   juice

1 egg, lightly beaten

50g/1¾ oz coconut oil, melted

2 tbsp agave syrup or honey

1–2 tbsp porridge (oatmeal) oats
   (gluten-free)

Prep 15 minutes / **Cooking** 30 minutes / **Makes** 1 large loaf

Heat the oven to 180°C/160°C fan/350°F/gas 4. Lightly oil a 900g/ 2 lb loaf tin.

Combine the flour, bicarbonate of soda, cinnamon and salt in a mixing bowl. Stir in the apple, apricots, your chosen nuts and the sunflower or pumpkin seeds.

Mix together the apple or cranberry juice, egg, coconut oil and agave syrup or honey, then pour into the bowl. Gently mix together, making sure you don't overmix so you have a lighter loaf.

Spoon into the prepared tin and scatter the oats over the top. Bake for 30 minutes, or until the top is lightly golden and a skewer comes out clean when inserted in the middle of the loaf. Cool in the tin for 10 minutes before serving warm or turning onto a wire rack to cool.

Flexible

Vegan: mix together 1 tablespoon ground flaxseed with 3 tablespoons cold water. Sit for 10 minutes to allow to thicken and use to replace the egg.

Flavour swap: you can swap the dried fruits and nuts in this loaf to suit your preferences. Dried cranberries, cherries, apple, dates, figs, sultanas (golden raisins) and raisins are all good. Grated pears can be used instead of the apples, and pretty much any fruit juice can be used.

Potato naan bread

An alternative to the usual flour naan bread, these brilliant breads use mashed potato and gram (chickpea) flour, both of which are gluten-free and suitable for vegans. They're delicious served warm with your favourite curry dishes to mop up any sauce.

For a lighter textured naan, it's best to go for a floury potato such as Désirée, Maris Piper or King Edward.

650g/1lb 2 oz potatoes, peeled
1 tsp caster (superfine) sugar
1 tbsp nigella (black onion) seeds
2 tsp onion granules
2 tsp flaked sea salt
1 tsp ground coriander
125g/4½ oz/scant 1 cup gram (chickpea) flour, plus extra for dusting
sunflower oil, for brushing

Prep 35 minutes / **Cooking** 35 minutes / **Makes** 6

Place the potatoes in a pan of boiling salted water for about 15–20 minutes until they are tender and cooked through. Reserve 100ml/3½ fl oz/scant ½ cup of the cooking liquid, then drain the remaining water from the potatoes. Leave to cool for about 10 minutes.

Heat the oven to 180°C/160°C fan/350°F/gas 4. Line two baking trays with baking parchment.

Mash the potatoes in a bowl until they are really smooth. Mix in the sugar, nigella seeds, onion granules, salt and coriander, then add the flour. Bring everything together by hand until you have a smooth, pliable but slightly sticky dough. If it is too dry at this point add some of the reserved potato cooking water.

Turn the dough out onto a worktop lightly dusted with gram flour. Divide into 6 pieces and shape each one into an oval or circle shape, around 1cm/½ inch thick. Place the naans on the baking trays and brush the tops with oil. Bake for 30–35 minutes until they are slightly puffed up and lightly golden. Cool for a few minutes before eating.

Flexible

Flavour swap: if you want to transform these into **Italian flatbreads**, swap the nigella (black onion) seeds, onion granules and ground coriander for 1 tablespoon chopped rosemary, 1 crushed garlic clove and 2 tablespoons finely chopped pitted black or green olives.

And for **Middle Eastern flatbreads**, use 1 tablespoon toasted sesame seeds, 1 teaspoon dried sumac and 1 teaspoon ground cumin instead of the nigella seeds, onion granules and ground coriander.

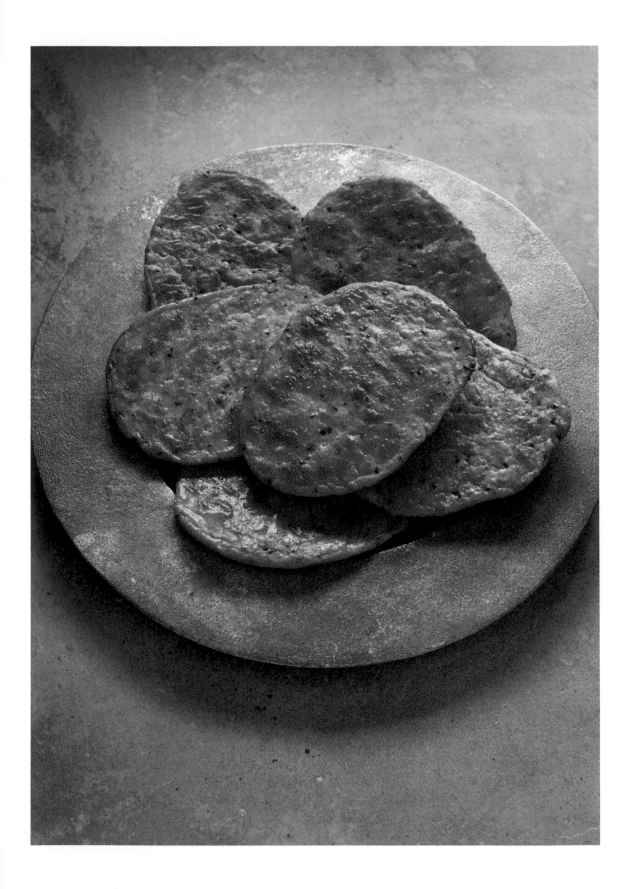

Basic white loaf

Sometimes all you want is a simple loaf of freshly baked bread. There really is very little that can prevent you from immediately wanting to tuck in as soon as this comes out from the oven. How you eat it is a personal choice – for me it has to be thickly sliced and spread with a delicious salted butter, and I'll always go back for a second slice!

1½ tsp flaked sea salt

400g/14 oz/3 cups strong white bread flour, plus extra for dusting

7g/2¼ tsp fast-action dried yeast

30g/1 oz butter, softened

olive or sunflower oil, for greasing

Prep 20 minutes, plus 2 hours rising / **Cooking** 30 minutes / **Makes** 1 large or 2 small loaves

Put the salt in the bottom of the bowl of an electric mixer fitted with a dough hook. Add the flour, then scatter over the yeast. Doing this will prevent the salt and yeast coming into contact before adding any liquid, as salt can slow down or even kill the yeast. Turn the mixer on to a slow speed and add the butter and 250ml/ 9 fl oz/1 cup lukewarm water. As the flour comes away from the side of the bowl, increase the speed to medium to knead the dough for about 5 minutes. If you feel the dough is too dry, add a little more water. You are after a soft smooth elastic dough.

Alternatively, if you don't have a machine, you can bring everything together in a large bowl and once you have a rough dough, turn onto a lightly oiled worktop and knead by hand for 10 minutes.

Transfer the dough to a large lightly oiled bowl and cover the bowl with a piece of oiled cling film. Leave to rise in a warm place for around 1 hour or more until it's at least doubled in size.

Lightly oil a 900g/2 lb loaf tin or two small 450g/1 lb tins.

Tip the risen dough onto a lightly floured surface. If you're making two loaves, divide the dough in half. Knock out the air by folding inwards on itself and creating a ball. Shape into a rectangle by flattening the dough slightly and bring the sides up to the middle. Turn over and sit in the loaf tin, with any seam underneath and a smooth surface on top. Cover loosely with oiled cling film or a large clean plastic bag. Leave to rise for a further 1 hour or so until doubled in size. The risen dough should spring back quickly if you prod it with your finger.

Heat the oven to 220°C/200°C fan/475°F/gas 7 and put a deep roasting tray on the bottom shelf to heat up.

When the dough has risen, dust the top/s lightly with flour. Half fill the roasting tray with boiling water to create steam, then put the loaf tin(s) on the shelf above. Bake for 20 minutes in small tins, or 30 minutes in the larger tin, or until golden and cooked. To check, tap the base of the loaf and it should sound hollow. Turn out of the tin and cool on a wire rack before slicing.

Flexible

Wholemeal loaf: *use 350g / 12 oz / 2½ cups strong wholemeal (wholewheat) bread flour and 50g / 1¾ oz / ⅓ cup strong white bread flour and continue with the recipe as above. You may need 1–2 tablespoons more water as wholemeal (wholewheat) flour absorbs more liquid.*

Bread rolls: *instead of making a single loaf, divide the dough into 8–10 pieces after the first rise. Shape into smooth balls and sit on a baking tray spaced slightly apart. Cover loosely with lightly oiled cling film or a large plastic bag and leave to rise until doubled, for about 1 hour. When risen, sprinkle with flour and bake as above for 15–20 minutes until golden. For a soft crust, don't put the water in the roasting tray in the oven.*

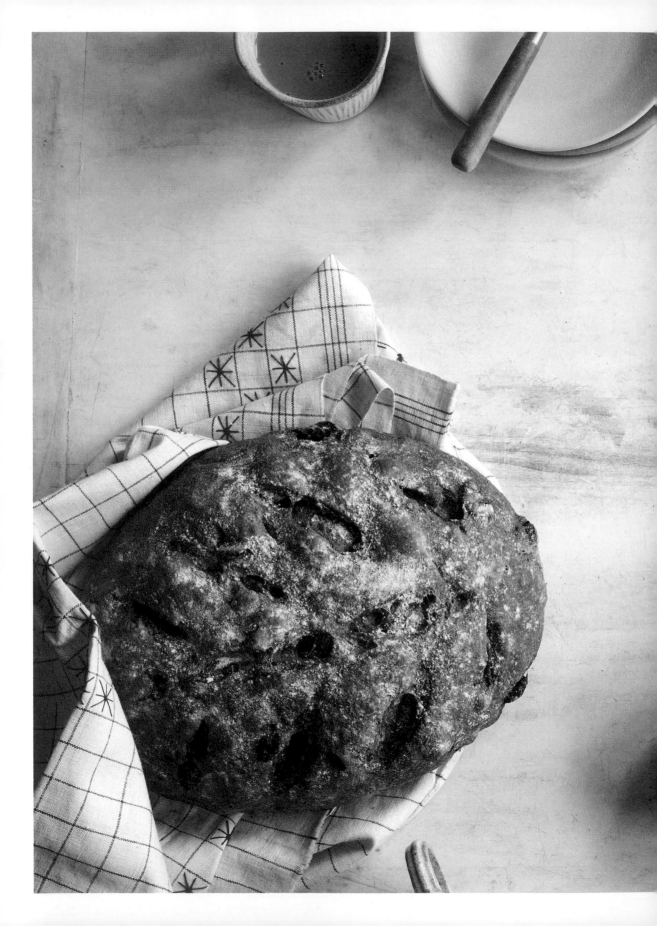

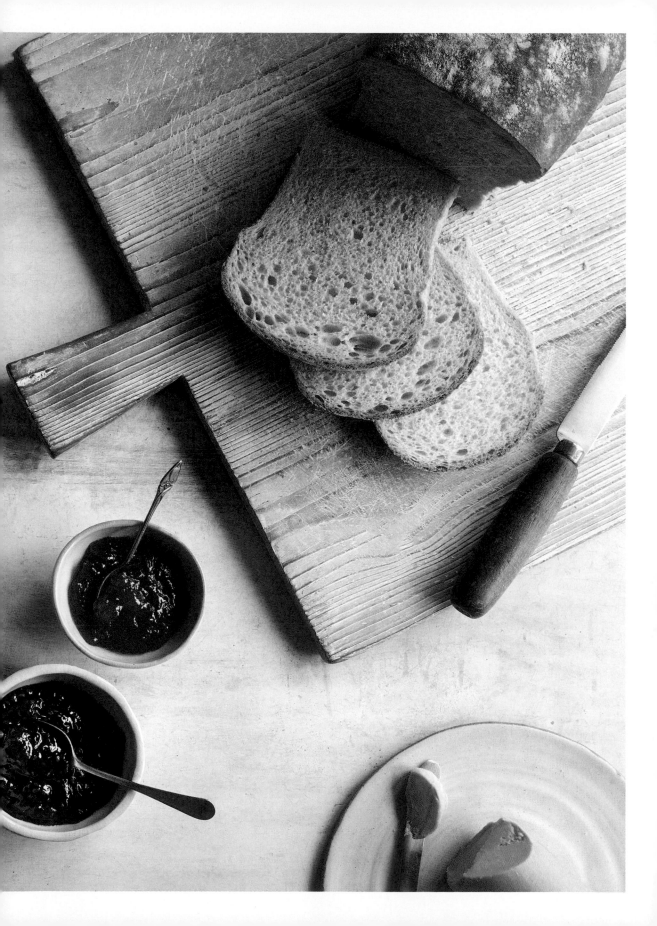

Walnut and raisin bread

This rustic loaf is brimming with flavour from the rye flour, sweet raisins, treacle and plenty of walnuts. Once made, it will last for days without going dry, in fact the flavour seems to become more intense from the day after it's made. It's particularly good served with strong cheeses, or even toasted for breakfast topped with ricotta and fresh figs, and drizzled with honey.

200g/7oz/1½ cups strong white bread flour, plus extra for dusting

200g/7oz/1½ cups strong wholemeal (wholewheat) bread flour

100g/3½ oz/¾ cup rye flour

2 tsp flaked sea salt

10g/¼ oz fast-action dried yeast

2 tbsp olive oil or walnut oil, plus extra for greasing

1 tbsp black treacle (molasses)

200g/7 oz/1½ cups walnut pieces, roughly chopped

150g/5½ oz/generous 1 cup raisins

Prep 20 minutes, plus 2 hours rising / **Cooking** 40 minutes / **Makes** 1 large loaf

Mix together the flours to combine. Put the salt in the bottom of the bowl of an electric mixer fitted with a dough hook. Tip the flours on top of the salt, then add the yeast, oil and treacle. Turn the mixer on to a slow speed and slowly add 325ml/11 fl oz/generous 1¼ cups lukewarm water. Increase the speed to medium to knead the dough for 5 minutes. If doing this by hand, knead on a lightly floured worktop for 8–10 minutes. If you feel the dough is too dry, add a little more water. You are after a soft texture but not too sticky.

Add the walnuts and raisins to the dough and mix in. Cover the bowl with a piece of lightly oiled cling film and leave to rise in a warm place for around 1 hour or until it's at least doubled in size.

Line a baking tray with baking parchment.

Transfer the risen dough onto a lightly floured surface and fold inwards on itself to knock out the air and make sure the dough is smooth. Shape into a loaf shape – round or oval, it's up to you. Sit on the baking tray. If you've a large clean plastic bag big enough, slide the tray inside, alternatively, use a large piece of oiled cling film to loosely cover the tray. Leave to rise for another 1 hour or so until doubled in size.

Heat the oven to 200°C/180°C fan/400°F/gas 6.

When the dough has risen, use a sharp knife to slash a pattern on the top and dust lightly with flour. Bake for 35–40 minutes until deep golden and sounds hollow when the base is tapped. Cool on a wire rack before slicing.

Flexible

Nut-free: *to make this into a fruit bread, omit the walnuts and use a 250g/ 9 oz / 1¾ cups combination of mixed dried fruits, such as raisins, sultanas (golden raisins), cherries, cranberries, chopped apricots or chopped dates.*

Flavour swap: *you can mix up the fruit and nut pairings to suit your own tastes. I like to use 200g/7 oz/2 cups chopped pecan nuts and 150g/5½ oz/ generous 1 cup dried cranberries around Christmas time, or 200g/7 oz/2 cups walnuts and 150g/5½ oz/1 cup chopped dried figs are a favourite to serve with cheese.*

'Sourdough' for the impatient

I love eating sourdough, but seldom have the patience for the full processes involved. So, I had a play around with various quick versions and finally came up with this recipe. The flavour and texture are fantastic – the main difference is that it does contain some yeast, which real sourdough doesn't, but if you are impatient like me, I highly recommend giving this a go.

200g/7 oz/1½ cups strong white bread
   flour, plus extra for dusting
200g/7 oz/1½ cups rye flour
1 tsp fast-action dry yeast
375g/13 oz/1¾ cups natural bio yoghurt
1½ tsp flaked sea salt
Vegetable oil, for greasing

Prep 20 minutes, plus up to 6 hours rising / **Cooking** 45 minutes / **Makes** 1 large loaf

Put the flours, yeast and yoghurt in the bowl of an electric mixer fitted with a dough hook. Sprinkle over the salt and mix together until a dough forms. Alternatively, if you don't have a mixer, you can put everything put in a large bowl and bring together by hand. Continue to knead for a good few minutes until the dough is smooth and springy but still quite sticky to touch.

Transfer to a large clean lightly oiled bowl and cover with a piece of oiled cling film and a warm damp cloth over the top for extra insulation. Leave the dough to ferment and rise at room temperature, until the dough has pretty much doubled in size. This should take about 4 hours.

Dust the worktop with some flour and turn the dough out of the bowl, taking care not to knock out all the air bubbles. Think of the dough as having four sides and fold the top third into the middle, then the bottom third over the top (a little like folding a letter), turn the dough a quarter turn and repeat the fold. This will help create some bigger air bubbles and texture to the finished bread. Shape into a round or oval shape smoothing the dough with your hands and transfer to a large piece of baking parchment dusted with flour – I find placing a baking tray under the parchment useful in case I need to move the dough during this proving stage. Place a large clean bowl over the top and leave for an hour or so to prove, and almost double in size again.

Heat the oven to 220°C/200°C fan/425°F/gas 7. Place a large, lidded casserole dish in the oven to heat up – make sure to use one that's big enough to fit the loaf in.

Once the dough has risen, take a very sharp knife and cut a deep slash on the top of the loaf, or do a few, to create your own unique pattern, and dust the top with some flour.

Remove the casserole dish from the oven and carefully lift the dough, still on the parchment, directly into the dish. Cover with the lid and bake in the oven for 30 minutes, before removing the lid and cooking for a further 10–15 minutes until the crust is deep golden and crisp.

Lift from the casserole dish and cool on a wire rack before slicing.

Flexible

Vegan: *the natural bio yoghurt can be swapped for a plant-based natural yoghurt with live dairy-free cultures. I like to use a natural coconut yoghurt made with live cultures, which gives a really delicious flavour when cooked.*

Flavour swap: *for a seeded sourdough, stir 2 tablespoons poppy, sesame or nigella (black onion) seeds into the flour at the start. Bake as on page 53.*

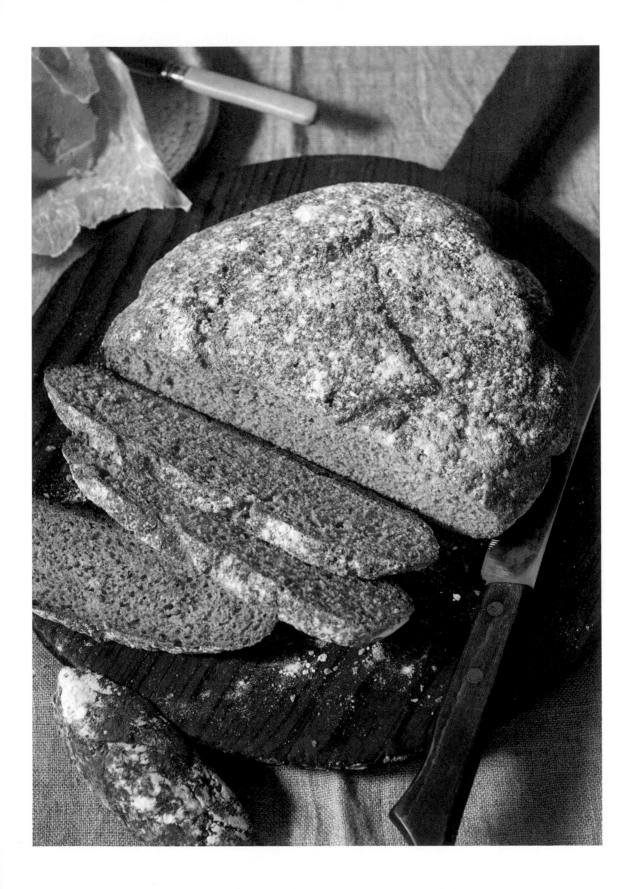

Parmesan grissini

*The number of times I have bought
breadsticks for a pre-dinner nibble
or snack for the kids is ludicrous,
but I had never thought about making
my own up until writing this book.
I played around with a few ideas for
traditional flour ones and gluten-free
versions and decided that the gluten-
free ones were the best to feature as the
main recipe as they are just so good.
They are easy to make and last for
days once made.*

200g/7 oz/1½ cups rice flour
100g/3½ oz/1 cup ground almonds
10g/½ oz cornflour (cornstarch)
7g/2¼ tsp fast-action dried yeast
1 tsp flaked sea salt
1 tsp xanthan gum
25g/1 oz finely grated Parmesan cheese
150ml/5 fl oz/⅔ cup milk
100g/3½ oz/½ cup butter, softened
1–2 tbsp flavourings such as poppy seeds,
   sesame seeds, nigella (black onion)
   seeds, finely chopped rosemary or
   thyme (optional)

Prep 30 minutes / **Cooking** 15 minutes / **Makes** 20

Heat the oven to 200°C/180°C fan/400°F/gas 6. Line a couple of
baking trays with baking parchment.

Put all of the ingredients, apart from the optional flavourings, into
an electric mixer with a dough hook. Alternatively, if you don't have
a mixer, place in a bowl and use your hands to form a ball of dough.
Knead the dough in the mixer, or by hand on the worktop for a few
minutes until you have a smooth dough.

Take pieces of dough, the size of a walnut, and roll into lengths
around 1cm/½ inch thick and around 20–25cm/8–10 inches long.

Now you can add any of the flavourings, if you are using them,
by scattering seeds or herbs over the work surface and rolling the
grissini over them so they stick.

Lay the grissini on the prepared baking trays, leaving a small gap
between each one, and bake for 12–15 minutes or until golden
brown. Leave to cool for a few minutes before enjoying warm when
they will still be a little soft, or they can be enjoyed over the next
few days when they will be firmer and crunchier.

Flexible

Traditional flour breadsticks: *you can make these breadsticks
using a standard white flour. To do this, you'll need to swap the rice
flour, ground almonds, cornflour (cornstarch) and xanthan gum for
300g / 10½ oz / generous 2 cups strong white bread flour and increase
the milk to 175ml / 6 fl oz / ¾ cup. Make and bake as above.*

Vegan: *the recipe will work in the same way by substituting the milk,
butter and Parmesan for plant-based alternatives.*

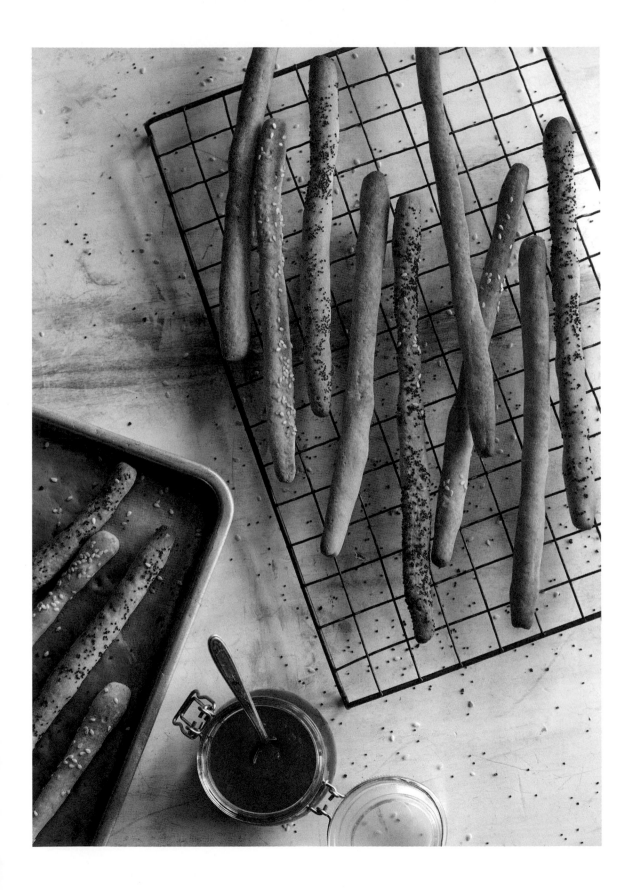

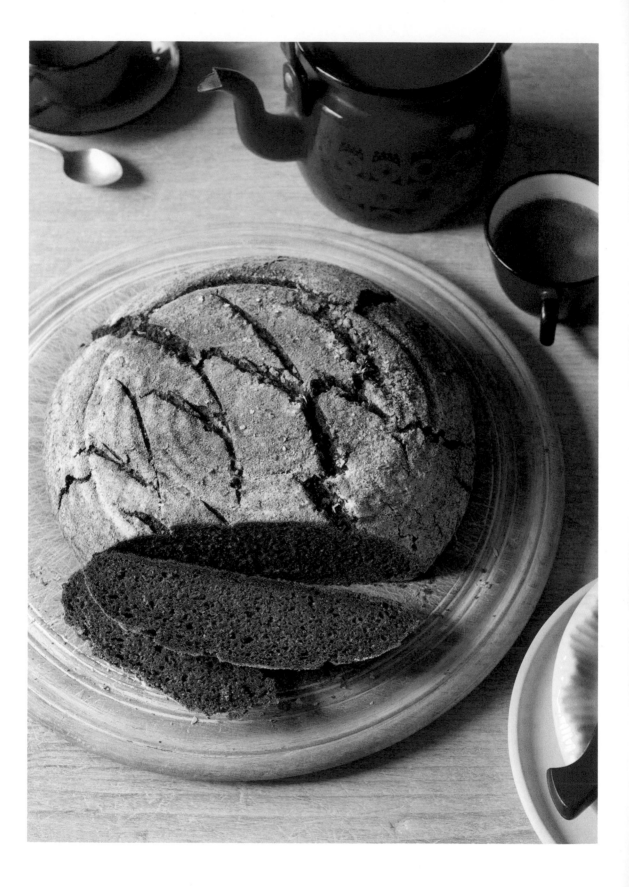

Rye bread

This one is a straightforward rye bread that has an earthy, nutty flavour from the rye flour and a rich sweetness from the treacle, although for variety you can try other flavours suggested in the Flexible section below.

Rye flour is lower in gluten than wheat flour, making the end result fairly dense, so it is best served in thin slices.

---

2 tsp flaked sea salt
500g/1 lb 2 oz/3⅔ cups rye flour, plus extra for dusting
10g/¼ oz fast-action dried yeast
1 tbsp black treacle (molasses)
oil, for greasing

Prep 20 minutes, plus 6 hours rising / **Cooking** 30 minutes / **Makes** 1 large loaf

Put the salt in the bottom of a large bowl, tip the flour on top, then scatter over the yeast.

In a small bowl, stir 250ml/9 fl oz/1 cup lukewarm water into the treacle and add this to the bowl, bringing the dough together with your fingers. Add a further 100ml/3½ fl oz/⅓ cup lukewarm water, a little at a time, until fully incorporated. You may not need all of the water – you want to end up with a soft moist dough that's not too sticky.

Lightly oil the worktop and turn out the dough. Knead for 5 minutes until smooth and the stickiness has gone. Sit the dough in a large, lightly oiled bowl, and cover with a damp tea towel. Leave to rise in a warm place for 3 hours until it's risen by around 1½ times its size.

Tip the dough onto a lightly floured surface and fold in on itself a few times to knock out the air. Shape into a smooth round ball, tucking the edges underneath. Generously dust a proving basket if you have one or lay a clean dry tea towel in a large bowl, and dust the tea towel generously with flour. Sit the dough smooth side down in the bowl and cover with a tea towel. Leave to prove for 2–3 hours, until it's risen by around 1½ times its size.

Heat the oven to 220°C/200°C fan/425°F/gas 7 and put a deep roasting tray on the bottom shelf to heat up.

Turn the risen dough onto a baking tray, floured side up. Slash a pattern on the top with a sharp knife. Half fill the roasting tray with boiling water then immediately put the bread on a shelf above it and close the door. Bake for 30 minutes. To check it's cooked, tap the base – it should sound hollow. Cool on a wire rack before slicing.

Flexible

Flavour swap: to make a **seeded rye bread**, you can add 100g/3½ oz/¾ cup sunflower or pumpkin seeds to the bowl before adding the water. Alternatively, for a chewier texture use 50g–100g/1¾ –3½ oz cracked rye to the flour.

To make **fruit and nut rye bread**, add 50g/1¾ oz/⅓ cup raisins and 75g/2¾ oz/½ cup roughly chopped walnuts into the bowl before adding the water.

Chipotle and Cheddar cornbread

Cornbread is a fantastic bread that's naturally gluten-free and very open to additional flavours. Here, I've added a burst of smoky spice from the chipotle paste, tangy bite from mature Cheddar cheese and a pop of sweetness from sweetcorn. It's a meal in itself, although would be great to serve with a bowl of tomato soup or steaming chilli.

200g/7 oz/1¼ cups polenta (cornmeal)

150g/5½ oz/1 cup gram (chickpea) flour

2 tbsp soft light brown sugar

1 tsp baking powder (gluten-free)

1 tsp flaked sea salt

½ tsp bicarbonate of (baking) soda

175g/6 oz mature Cheddar cheese, grated

285g/10 oz/2 cups sweetcorn, drained
 if tinned

4 spring onions (scallions), finely sliced

300ml/10 fl oz/scant 1½ cups soured
 cream

2 eggs, beaten

125ml/4 fl oz/½ cup olive oil, plus extra
 for drizzling

1½ tbsp chipotle paste

Prep 20 minutes, plus cooling / **Cooking** 35 minutes / **Serves** 6–8

Heat the oven to 200°C/180°C fan/400°F/gas 6. Line a 20cm/8 inch square cake tin (or similar size whether rectangular or round) with baking parchment.

Put the polenta, gram flour, sugar, baking powder, salt and bicarbonate of soda in a large mixing bowl and mix together until combined. Reserve about 50g/1¾ oz of the cheese and stir the rest into the bowl until it's coated in the floury mix.

In a separate bowl, mix together the sweetcorn, spring onions, soured cream, eggs, olive oil and chipotle paste until combined. Pour this into the cheese mix and stir until everything is just mixed together.

Spoon into the prepared tin, level the surface with the back of the spoon, and scatter over the remaining cheese. Drizzle over a little oil and bake in the oven for 30–35 minutes, until the top is golden, the centre firm and springy to touch and if a skewer is inserted in the middle, it comes out clean.

Once cooked, cool in the tin for about 20 minutes before removing and serving warm or cold. This is best eaten on the day of baking. Any leftovers can be frozen and gently warmed through in the oven.

Flexible

Vegan: *to make this into a vegan cornbread there are a few simple changes. Firstly, swap the cheese for a plant-based alternative. Instead of soured cream, you can use a plant-based natural yoghurt, or stir 1 tablespoon lemon juice into 300ml / 10 fl oz / 1¼ cups plant-based milk and leave to sit for 5 minutes to thicken before using. Finally, as an alternative to the eggs, mix together 2 tablespoons ground flaxseed with 6 tablespoons cold water. Sit for 2 minutes and add to the mixture as above.*

Flavour swap: *the addition of 6 finely sliced rashers of smoked streaky bacon, that have been fried until golden and added to the cornbread mix when adding the cheese, is delicious. Equally, you can add some finely diced chorizo or salami if you prefer.*

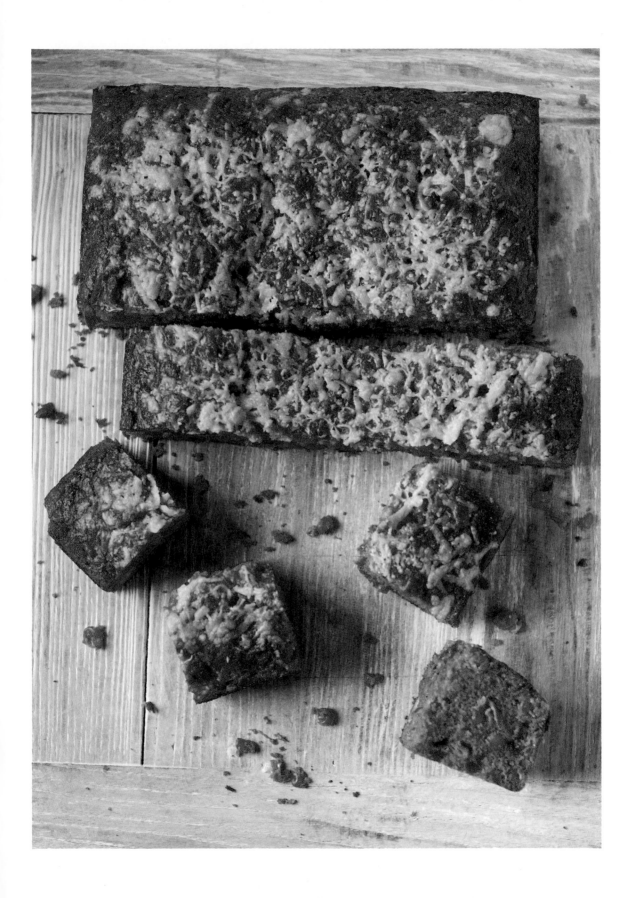

Spelt and prune tea loaf

This is a combination of a loaf and a cake, due to its light texture. It's packed with wholesome goodness, and is delicious on its own or spread with a little butter at breakfast, as an afternoon treat or in a lunchbox. Once made, it will last a good few days in an airtight container or can be frozen for up to 3 months.

100g/3½ oz/¾ cup prunes, chopped

50ml/2 fl oz/¼ cup strong black tea, hot

3 tbsp rapeseed (canola), sunflower
  or olive oil

1 egg, beaten

50g/1¾ oz/ ¼ cup natural yoghurt

50g/1¾ oz/ ¼ cup honey

2 tsp black treacle (molasses)

150g/5½ oz/1 cup wholemeal (whole)
  spelt flour

1 tsp bicarbonate of (baking) soda

1 tbsp demerara (turbinado) sugar

Prep 25 minutes / **Cooking** 35 minutes / **Makes** 1 small loaf

Heat the oven to 180°C/160°C fan/350°F/gas 4. Line a 450g/1 lb loaf tin with baking parchment, or if it is non-stick, just rub a little oil around the inside.

Put the prunes in a small bowl and pour over the tea. Leave to soak for 10 minutes.

In a large bowl, beat together the oil, egg, yoghurt, honey and treacle until you have a smooth batter. Add the flour and bicarbonate of soda, then mix well. Finally, stir in the prunes and any remaining tea that hasn't soaked into the prunes.

Spoon the mixture into the loaf tin and scatter over the demerara sugar. Bake for 35 minutes or until a skewer comes out clean when inserted in the centre of the loaf.

Cool in the tin for 10 minutes before transferring to a wire rack to cool completely.

Flexible

Gluten-free: you can do a straight swap and use buckwheat flour instead of spelt flour.

Vegan: as a vegan alternative to 1 egg, mix 1 tablespoon ground flaxseed with 3 tablespoons cold water and leave to thicken for 10 minutes, use in the same way as the egg. A plant-based unsweetened yoghurt can be swapped for the natural yoghurt, and use agave or maple syrup instead of honey.

*Flavour swap: for a festive **Christmas loaf**, use whisky instead of tea and add ½ teaspoon mixed (apple pie) spice and the finely grated zest of ½ orange to the mixture.*

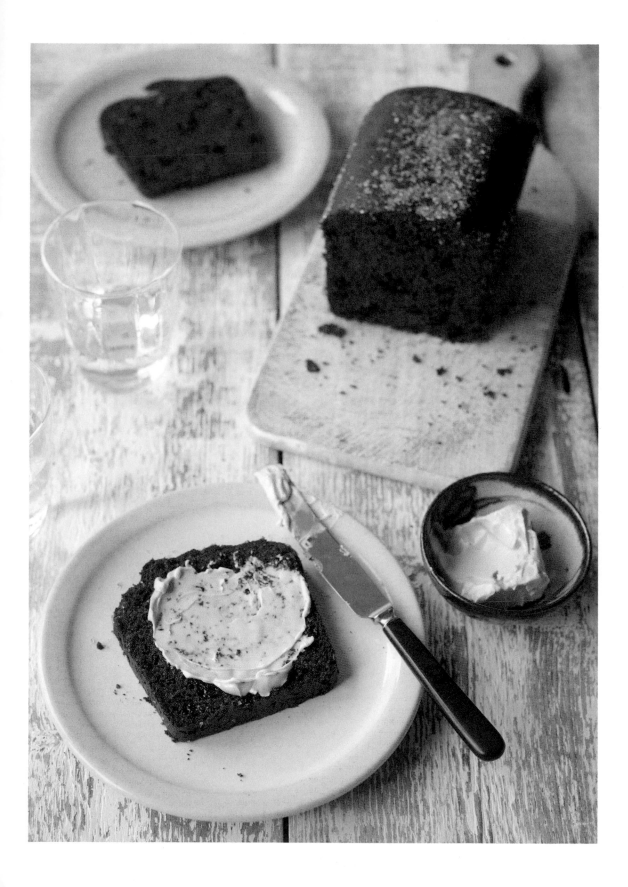

Sticky cinnamon rolls

This might seem like a lengthy recipe but it's surprisingly straightforward to make and great to get stuck into with children. To get ahead, you can prepare the cinnamon rolls up to the point of placing them in the tin and keep the tin covered in the fridge overnight. Return to room temperature for about 30 minutes and bake as per the recipe, giving you soft, freshly baked cinnamon rolls on the day you're wanting to eat them.

For the rolls

175ml/6fl oz/¾ cup milk

7g/2¼ tsp fast-action dried yeast

50g/1¾ oz/¼ cup caster (superfine) sugar

1 egg and 1 egg yolk, beaten

40g/1½ oz butter, melted, plus extra
  for greasing

450g/1 lb/3¼ cups strong white bread
  flour, plus extra for dusting

½ tsp fine sea salt

For the filling

125g/4½ oz/½ cup butter, softened

100g/3½ oz/½ cup soft dark brown sugar

1½ tbsp ground cinnamon

For the syrup

50g/1¾ oz/¼ cup caster (superfine) sugar

½ tsp ground cinnamon

For the glaze

50g/1¾ oz/⅓ cup icing (confectioners')
  sugar

Prep 20 minutes, plus 2 hours rising / **Cooking** 25 minutes /
Makes 9

Gently heat the milk until it's lukewarm, around 40°C/100°F. Transfer to the bowl of an electric mixer fitted with a dough hook. Mix in the yeast, sugar, eggs and melted butter, then add the flour and salt. Mix until you have a sticky dough, then knead for around 5 minutes in the mixer until you have a smooth elastic dough.

Transfer to a large lightly oiled bowl, cover with a damp tea towel or oiled cling film and leave to rise in a warm place for 1–1½ hours or until doubled in size.

Lightly grease a square baking tin, roughly 20 x 30cm/8 x 12 inches with butter and line the base with baking parchment. Turn the dough out onto a floured worktop. Roll out into a 20 x 27cm/8 x 10 inch rectangle, with the longer edges being at the top and bottom, shorter edges at the sides.

Combine the filling ingredients, then spread over the dough leaving 1cm/½ inch at the top edge. Tightly roll the dough away from you, making a long sausage with the seam underneath. Cut into 9 slices and place cut side up in the tin, leaving space between them to rise. Cover loosely with oiled cling film and leave in a warm place to rise for 30 minutes.

Heat the oven to 180°C/160°C fan/350°F/gas 4. Bake for about 20–25 minutes, until lightly golden.

To make the syrup, add the sugar, cinnamon and 3 tablespoons water to a small saucepan and gently heat until it starts to simmer. To make the glaze, mix 2 tablespoons water into the icing sugar until smooth. Liberally brush the hot cinnamon rolls with the hot syrup. Cool in the tin then remove and drizzle over the glaze.

Flexible

*For **festive buns**, scatter 25g / 1 oz melted butter, 75g / 2¾ oz / ⅓ cup soft brown sugar, 2 teaspoons ground mixed (apple pie) spice, 100g / 3½ oz / ¾ cup dried cranberries and 100g / 3½ oz / ¾ cup finely chopped dried apricots over the dough in place of the cinnamon mix. Roll and bake as above. Glaze with 100g / 3½ oz / ¾ cup icing (confectioners') sugar mixed with 1 tablespoon orange juice and finely grated zest of ½ orange.*

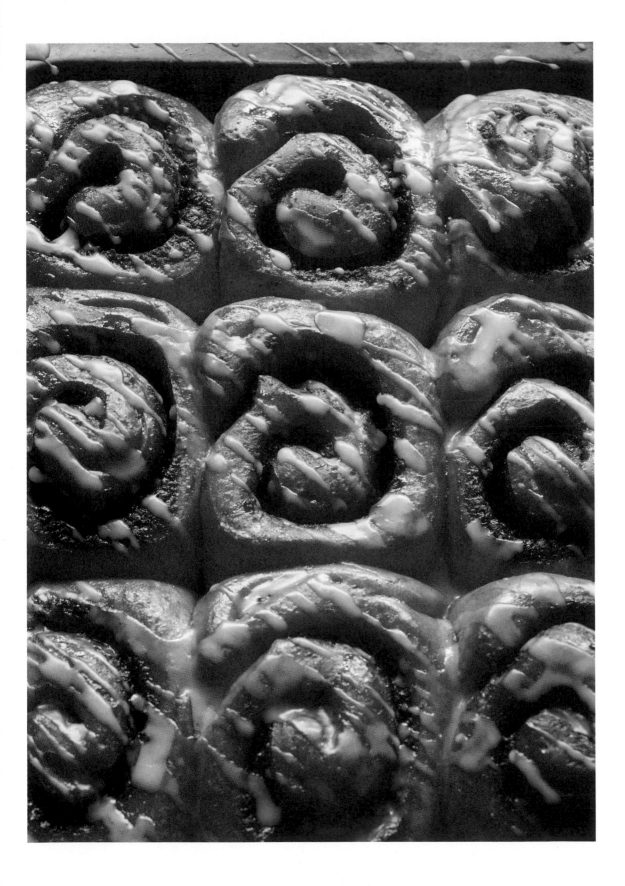

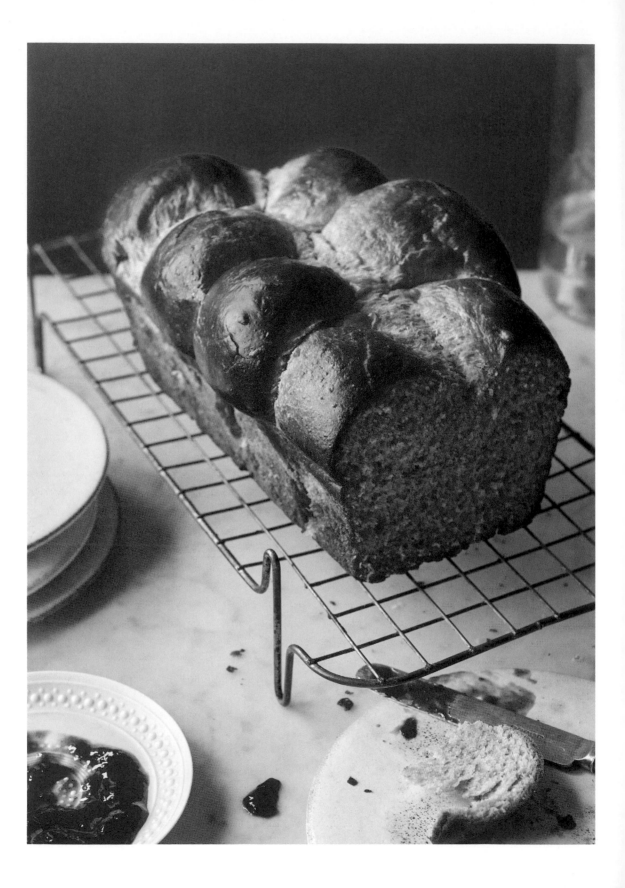

Brioche

Out of all the bread recipes I make at home, this one has to be the most popular with the kids, where they will plaster it thickly with chocolate spread. Not the healthiest of choices but it's not a bread you'd make every day. The egg and butter in the dough make this rich, but amazingly light in texture. You'll need a mixer with a dough hook for this recipe to make sure the soft butter mixes in properly. Once the dough is made, it has to chill overnight making it easier to shape into the classic brioche loaf. The preparation time required is well worth it as believe me, once baked you will be super impressed with your homemade brioche loaf.

75ml/5 tbsp/⅓ cup milk

40g/1½ oz/scant ¼ cup caster (superfine) sugar

1 tsp fine sea salt

300g/10½ oz/2 cups strong white bread flour, plus extra for dusting

7g/2¼ tsp fast-action dried yeast

3 eggs, beaten, plus 1 extra, beaten, for glazing

125g/4½ oz/½ cup butter, diced and softened

Prep 40 minutes, plus overnight resting and 1 hour rising / **Cooking** 35 minutes / **Makes** 1 large loaf

Gently heat the milk until it is lukewarm. If you have a thermometer, it needs to be around 40°C/100°F. Stir in the sugar until it's dissolved.

Put the salt in the bottom of the bowl of an electric mixer fitted with a dough hook. Add the flour, then scatter over the yeast. Set the machine to medium and pour in the milk, then gradually add the eggs, mixing for 10 minutes until you have a smooth elastic dough.

With the mixer running, add the butter a couple of pieces at a time, mixing until fully incorporated. Continue kneading the dough for a further 10 minutes, or until the dough is elastic and pulling away from the sides of the bowl. Tip the dough into a large lightly greased bowl. Cover with oiled cling film and leave in the fridge overnight.

Line the bottom and sides of a 900g/2 lb loaf tin with baking parchment. Remove the dough from the fridge and tip onto a worktop dusted with flour. Divide into 7 equal pieces and shape each one into a smooth ball.

Put the balls into the tin, four on one side and three in the gaps on the other side. Loosely cover with a clean tea towel and leave to rise in a warm place for about 1 hour, or until almost doubled in size.

Heat the oven to 180°C/160°C fan/350°F/gas 4. Brush the top of the risen dough with the remaining egg. Bake for 30–35 minutes until golden and risen. Leave to cool in the tin for 10 minutes before turning out onto a wire rack to cool completely.

Flexible

*Flavour swap: to make **chocolate brioche**, mix 150g/5½ oz dark chocolate chips into the dough just before chilling it in the fridge. Cook as above.*

*Add some festive flavour by making **'panettone' brioche**. Warm 3 tablespoons dark rum in a small pan and stir in 75g/2¾ oz/½ cup raisins and 75g/2¾ oz/½ cup candied peel. Remove from the heat and leave to soak for 1 hour. Mix into the dough before chilling it in the fridge. Cook as above, checking the top doesn't burn where any fruit is exposed. Cover lightly with foil if it appears to be.*

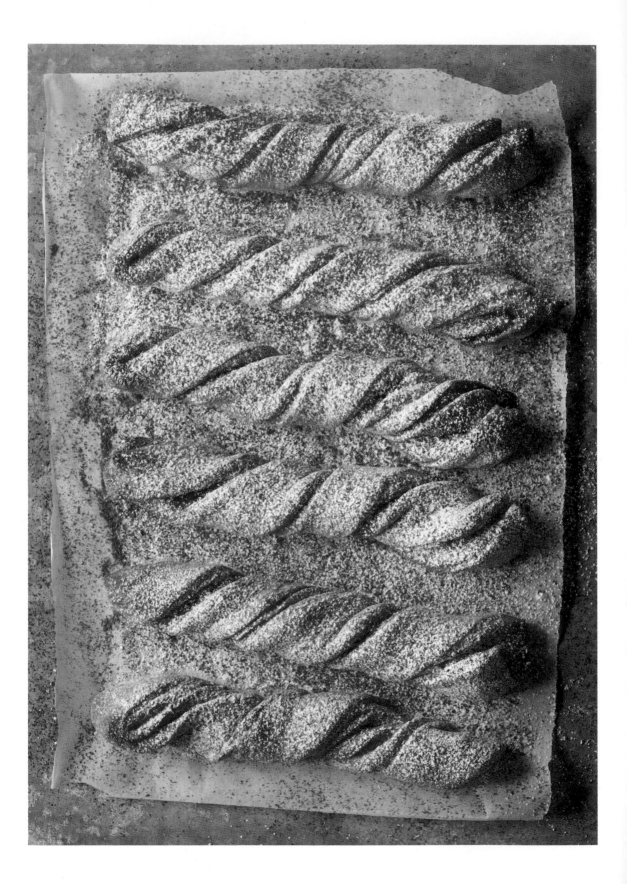

Raspberry twists

These tangy raspberry, soft dough twists not only look really impressive – they taste amazing, too. As with most homemade bread recipes, these are best eaten on the day of making and believe me they are very hard to resist, so that really won't be a problem. As a get-ahead tip for you, they can be put in the fridge for 24 hours once they have been shaped into twists. Before baking, leave them to rise for about 45 minutes (rather than the 25 minutes as stated in the recipe).

For the dough

500g/1 lb 2 oz/3¾ cups plain (all-purpose) flour, plus extra for dusting

7g/2¼ tsp fast-action dried yeast

50g/1¾ oz/¼ cup caster (superfine) sugar

200ml/7 fl oz/generous ¾ cup milk

50g/1¾ oz butter, softened

1 egg, beaten

½ tsp fine sea salt

oil, for greasing

For the filling

125g/4½ oz raspberry jam (jelly)

For the topping

25g/1 oz butter, melted

50g/1¾ oz/¼ cup caster (superfine) sugar

freeze-dried raspberry powder

icing (confectioners') sugar, for dusting

Prep 40 minutes, plus, 1¼ hours rising / **Cooking** 20 minutes / **Makes** 12

To make the dough, put about half of the flour in the bowl of an electric mixer fitted with a dough hook. Add the yeast and sugar. Stir to combine.

Heat the milk so it's lukewarm, around 40°C/100°F. Add to the bowl along with the butter, egg and salt. Mix until combined and very sticky, then add the remaining half of the flour.

Knead for 5 minutes until smooth and elastic. Transfer to a lightly oiled bowl and cover with a damp tea towel or oiled cling film. Leave to rise in a warm place for 50 minutes or until doubled in size.

Turn onto a floured surface and gently roll into a large rectangle, approximately 20 x 30cm/8 x 12 inches. Spread the jam over the surface, leaving a 2cm/¾ inch border. Fold in half lengthways and press the edges with the rolling pin to seal. Re-roll the dough, to give you a rectangle roughly the size you started with.

Cut the dough into 12 strips, 2.5cm/1 inch wide. Twist the strips as you place them down onto two baking trays lined with baking parchment, spacing slightly apart and loosely cover with oiled cling film. Leave to rest for around 25 minutes in a warm place.

Heat the oven to 180°C/160°C fan/350°F/gas 4.

Brush the raspberry twists with the melted butter and sprinkle generously with sugar. Bake for 20 minutes until light golden. As soon as they are out of the oven, sprinkle with freeze-dried raspberry powder and a dusting of icing sugar.

Flexible

*Flavour swap: to make **apricot and almond twists**, spread 125g/ 4½ oz apricot jam (jelly) over the rolled out dough and grate over 75g/ 2¾ oz marzipan. Fold and re-roll as per the recipe. Scatter over a few flaked (slivered) almonds on top of each twist before baking.*

*For **pecan and chocolate twists**, spread 125g/4½ oz chocolate spread over the rolled out dough and scatter over 75g/2¾ oz/¾ cup chopped pecan nuts. Once baked, sprinkle over some grated chocolate or a light dusting of cocoa powder.*

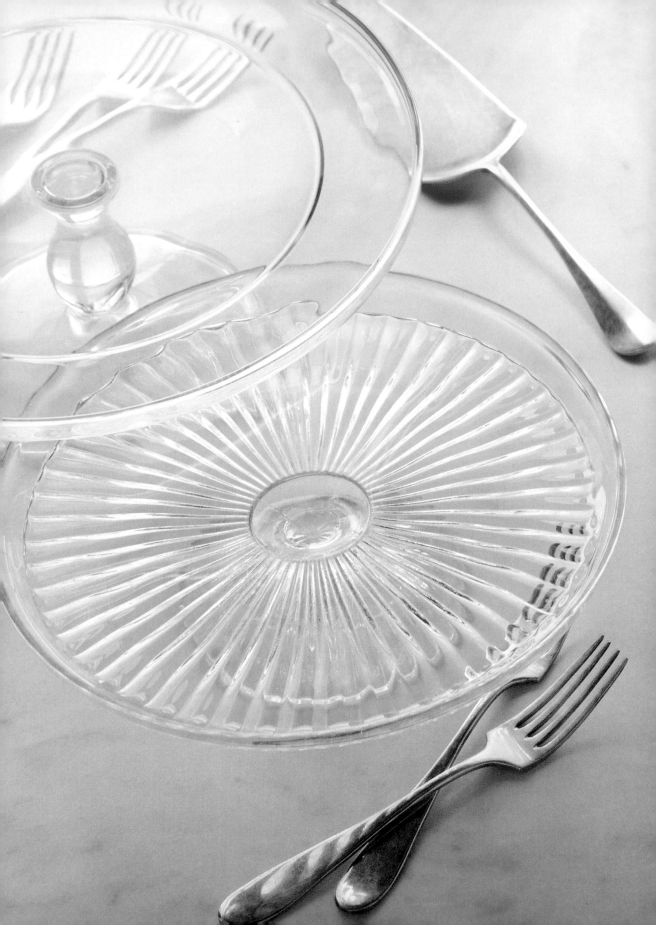

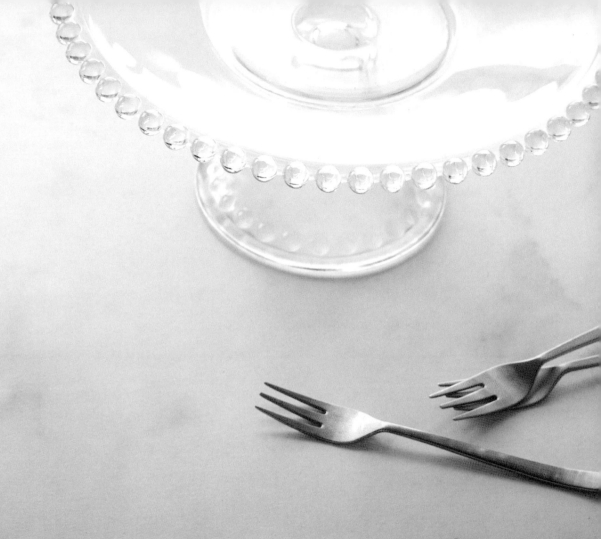

cakes and
traybakes

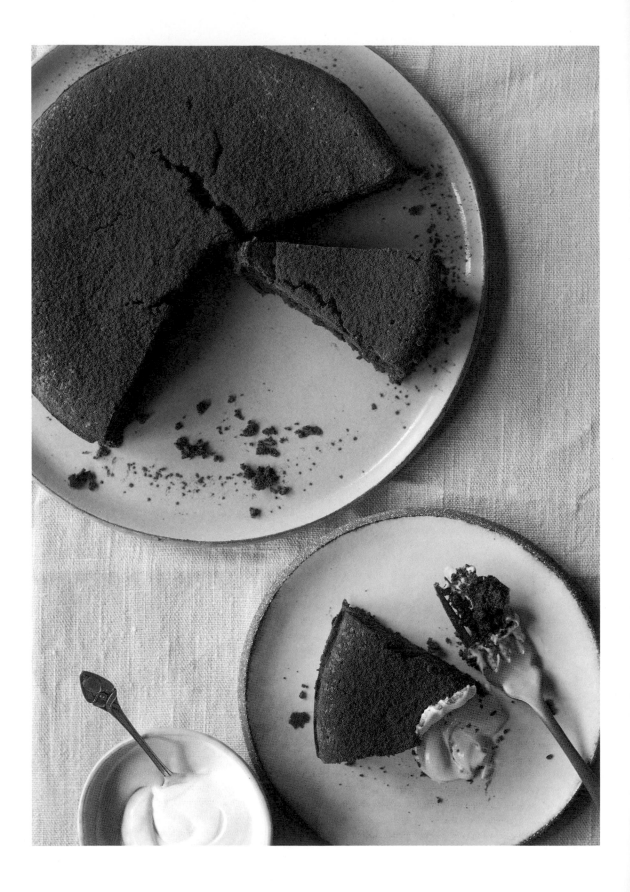

Rich chocolate truffle cake

This delightfully dense chocolate cake tends to be my go-to recipe when I need to make a quick-to-prepare, minimal fuss cake to serve as a dessert when entertaining. You can easily switch the flavour around depending on which liqueur is used – it's a very flexible cake.

Serve warm or chilled, just as it is or topped with berries or cherries and a dollop of crème fraîche or thick cream.

175g/6 oz dark chocolate
  (70 per cent cocoa solids), chopped
175g/6 oz/¾ cup butter, plus extra for
  greasing
175g/6 oz/scant 1 cup soft brown sugar
1 tsp vanilla bean paste
6 eggs
175g/6 oz/scant 2 cups ground almonds
2 tbsp of your chosen liqueur (optional)
  such as brandy, whisky, orange, almond,
  hazelnut, coconut or coffee
1 tbsp cocoa powder, for dusting

Prep 30 minutes / **Cooking** 40 minutes / **Serves** 8–10

Heat the oven to 180°C/160°C fan/350°F/gas 4. Grease a 20cm/ 8 inch cake tin with butter and line the base with baking parchment.

Place the chocolate in a bowl over a pan of barely simmering water to slowly melt. Alternatively, gently melt in the microwave in 10-second bursts.

Beat together the butter, sugar and vanilla using an electric mixer, until it's creamy and light in texture. Add the eggs, one at a time, beating well after each addition. Pour in the melted chocolate in a steady stream, beating as you pour, until combined and you have a creamy consistency.

Mix in the ground almonds and chosen liqueur, if using, then pour into the prepared tin, levelling out the surface.

Bake for 35–40 minutes until risen and just firm in the centre, with a very slight wobble.

Leave in the tin for 10 minutes before sliding a table knife around the inside edge of the tin and removing the cake altogether to cool on a wire rack.

Serve at room temperature for a softer texture, or if you want a firmer cake, then serve chilled. Dust the surface with cocoa powder just before serving.

Flexible

Nut-free: *the same weight of desiccated (shredded) coconut can be used as a nut-free alternative. However, you can also use the same weight of plain (all-purpose) flour, gluten-free flour blend or coconut flour.*

Dairy-free: *use a plant-based butter alternative or margarine. Coconut oil can also be used, which has a very distinctive taste and works really nicely with the addition of a coconut liqueur.*

Flavour swap: *if you don't want to use alcoholic liqueurs to add flavour, then you can add the finely grated zest of 1 orange, 1 teaspoon almond or coconut essence, 1 teaspoon orange blossom water or rosewater or 2 tablespoons very strong espresso coffee.*

Lemon and blackberry layer cake

Whether it's a celebration or just an afternoon treat, this cake is suitable for any occasion. Unlike standard butter-based sponges, this one is made with oil, which gives such a lovely moistness to the cake making it last a good few days rather than drying out.

This cake also comes with many flexible options, so you can swap around flavours to suit your tastes, occasion or season.

For the cake
200g/7 oz/1 cup caster (superfine) sugar
3 eggs
200g/7 oz/1½ cups self-raising (self-rising) flour
225g/8 oz/scant 1 cup sunflower oil, plus extra for greasing
150ml/5 fl oz/⅔ cup milk
finely grated zest of 2 lemons
½ tsp fine sea salt

For the compote
200g/7 oz/1½ cups blackberries, fresh or frozen (defrosted if frozen)
50g/1¾ oz/¼ cup caster (superfine) sugar
juice of 1 lemon
1 tsp arrowroot powder

For the buttercream
225g/8 oz/1 cup butter, softened
375g/13 oz/2⅔ cups icing (confectioners') sugar, sifted
2 tbsp milk
finely grated zest of 1 lemon

Prep 45 minutes / **Cooking** 25 minutes / **Serves** 12

Heat the oven to 180°C/160°C fan/350°F/gas 4. Brush two 20cm/8 inch loose-bottomed cake tins with oil and line with parchment.

To make the sponge, place the sugar and eggs in a mixing bowl and whisk until they are light in colour and frothy. Add the remaining ingredients. Stir until combined and pour into the cake tins.

Bake for 20–25 minutes until golden brown and the sponge is just coming away from the edge of the tins. Set aside to cool for 5 minutes, then run a palette knife around the inside edge of the tins. Carefully turn the cakes out onto a cooling rack to cool completely.

To make the blackberry compote, put the blackberries, sugar and lemon juice in a saucepan. Bring to a simmer and cook over a low–medium heat for 10 minutes or until the blackberries have broken down. Push through a sieve and return to a clean saucepan. Mix the arrowroot with 1 teaspoon water to form a paste. Stir into the purée and cook over a medium heat, stirring all the time until just simmering. Set aside to cool – it will thicken slightly as it cools.

Place the ingredients for the buttercream in a large bowl or the bowl of an electric mixer. Set your mixer to a low speed and gradually increase it until you have a smooth, creamy buttercream.

To assemble, place one cake upside down and spread it with some buttercream. Turn the other cake upside down and spread a generous layer of blackberry compote. Sandwich together. Spread a thick layer of buttercream on the top and sides of the cake, smoothing the edges with a palette knife (for a super smooth finish, dip the knife into hot water before you spread). Finish by swirling some compote through the buttercream on the top of the cake.

Flexible
__Gluten-free:__ swap the flour for a gluten-free flour blend and add an additional 50ml / 2 fl oz / scant ¼ cup milk to the cake batter.

__Dairy-free:__ use a non-dairy milk in the cake such as soya, almond or my favourite, fresh coconut milk. For the lemon buttercream, swap butter for a plant-based alternative (preferably a firm, not spreadable, one).

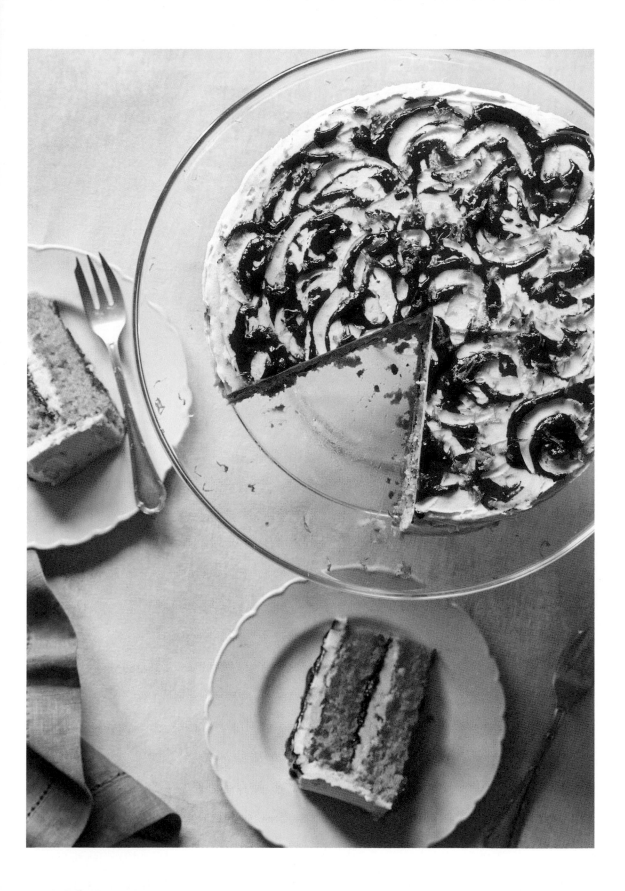

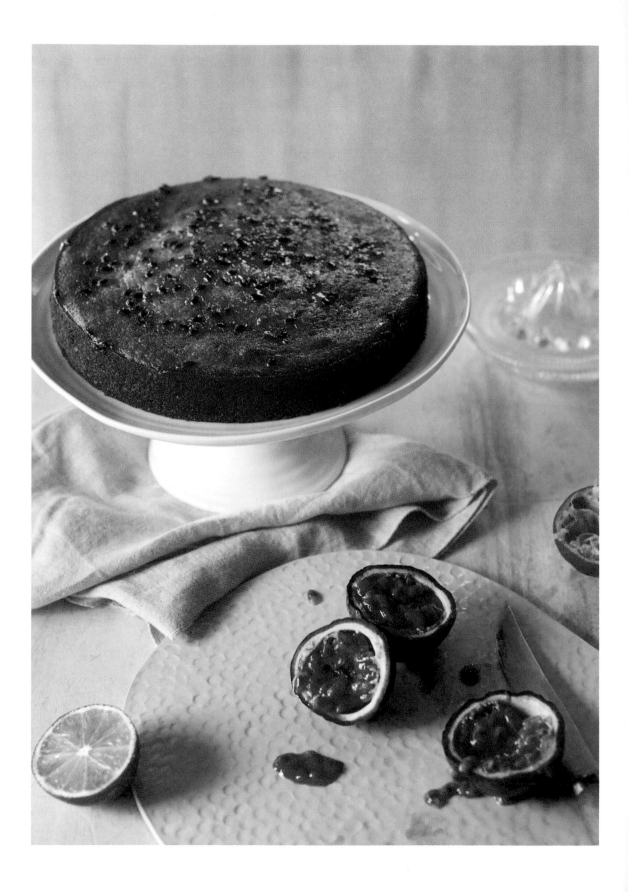

Sticky lime and passion fruit cake

Super tangy lime and sharp passion fruit are such a perfect match. In this recipe they feature both in the cake mixture and to create an absolutely delicious sticky syrup that's poured over the top once the cake is cooked.

This dairy-free cake can easily be transformed into a vegan treat by following the Flexible section below.

250g/9 oz/1¼ cups caster (superfine) sugar

finely grated zest and juice of 2 limes

3 ripe passion fruit

175ml/6 fl oz/¾ cup olive or rapeseed (canola) oil, plus extra for greasing

2 eggs

180g/6 oz/generous ¾ cup coconut yoghurt

2 tsp baking powder

180g/6 oz/1⅓ cups plain (all-purpose) flour

Prep 30 minutes / **Cooking** 45 minutes / **Serves** 8–10

Heat the oven to 180°C/160°C fan/350°F/gas 4. Brush a 20cm/ 8 inch round deep cake tin with some oil and line the base with baking parchment.

Put 100g/3½ oz/½ cup of the sugar in a small saucepan. Measure the lime juice and make up the quantity to 100ml/3½ fl oz/scant ½ cup with water. Put in the saucepan along with the pulp from one of the passion fruit, reserving the other two for the cake. Bring to the boil and cook for 2 minutes or so until you have a loose syrup. Remove from the heat and set aside.

Beat together the oil, the remaining 150g/5½ oz/¾ cup sugar, the eggs, coconut yoghurt, pulp from the remaining two passion fruit and reserved lime zest, to give you a thin batter consistency. Mix the baking powder into the flour, then stir into the batter. Pour into the prepared tin and level the surface with the back of your spoon.

Bake for 40–45 minutes until golden and a skewer comes out clean when inserted in the middle.

Once baked, slowly pour the syrup over the top of the cake while it's still hot, allowing it to soak in. Cool in the tin for 10 minutes before turning out onto a cooling rack to cool further. Serve warm or at room temperature.

Flexible

Vegan: *substitute the eggs for 2 tablespoons chia seeds mixed with 6 tablespoons cold water. Sit for 10 minutes until thickened before adding to the cake batter instead of the eggs in the above recipe.*

Flavour swap: *to make a **sticky blood orange cake**, swap the limes for 2 blood oranges when in season, and omit the passion fruit. Use Greek yoghurt (or almond yoghurt for dairy-free) instead of a coconut yoghurt.*

Chocolate cupcakes

Whether you are in the mood for something rich and chocolatey, or fresh and citrussy, these light springy cupcakes use oil rather than butter, so will keep moist and fresh for a good few days – ideal if you want to plan ahead for an occasion or celebration. Better still, as they contain no eggs or dairy, they should be your go-to recipe when you need to take dietary requirements into consideration. There are plenty of other flavour suggestions for you to try for each of the recipes in the Flexible sections below.

For the cakes
325ml/11 fl oz/1⅓ cups soya, oat, coconut or almond milk (avoid almond for nut-free)
2 tsp white wine vinegar or apple cider vinegar
225g/8 oz/1¾ cups self-raising (self-rising) flour
25g/1 oz cocoa powder
200g/7 oz/1 cup caster (superfine) sugar
100ml/3½ fl oz/scant ½ cup sunflower oil
1 tsp vanilla bean paste

For the frosting
50g/1¾ oz dark chocolate (dairy-free), chopped
150g/5½ oz plant-based margarine or butter
300g/10½ oz/2 cups icing (confectioners') sugar, sifted
1 tbsp soya, oat, coconut or almond milk
white, milk or dark chocolate (dairy-free) shavings or flakes, to decorate

Prep 30 minutes / **Cooking** 20 minutes / **Makes** 12

Heat the oven to 180°C/160°C fan/350°F/gas 4. Line a deep muffin tin with 12 muffin cases.

In a jug, stir the milk and vinegar together in a jug and leave to stand for a few minutes until the milk thickens and curdles slightly.

In a large bowl, sift together the flour and cocoa powder and stir in the sugar until combined. Whisk in the thickened milk as well as the oil and vanilla until you have a smooth loose batter.

Divide the batter between the muffin cases. I find this easier to do evenly with an ice-cream scoop although a jug or ladle are also good. The cases should be about two-thirds full.

Bake in the oven for 20 minutes until risen and golden. Turn the muffins out to cool on a wire rack.

To make the frosting, place the chocolate in a bowl over a pan of barely simmering water to slowly melt. Alternatively, gently melt in the microwave in 10-second bursts. Set aside to cool for 10 minutes.

In a large bowl, beat together the margarine or butter until smooth, then add the icing sugar and beat well until light and creamy. Add the melted chocolate and 1 tablespoon milk. Beat until totally mixed in then either pipe or spread over the top of the cupcakes. Decorate with some shavings or flakes of chocolate.

Flexible

*Flavour swap: to make **double chocolate orange cupcakes**, make the cake batter as above, adding the finely grated zest of 1 orange and 75g/2¾ oz dairy-free chocolate chips.*

*For a twist on the frosting, try a **chocolate caramel frosting**. Swirl 5 tablespoons vegan caramel through the chocolate frosting and pipe or spread onto the cupcakes. Finish with a drizzle of extra caramel on top (gently warmed first to loosen if necessary).*

Lemon and raspberry cupcakes

Prep 40 minutes / **Cooking** 20 minutes / **Makes** 12

Heat the oven to 180°C/160°C fan/350°F/gas 4. Line a deep muffin tin with 12 muffin cases.

In a jug, stir the milk and lemon juice together and leave to stand for a few minutes until the milk thickens and curdles slightly.

For the cakes

325ml/11 fl oz/1⅓ cups soya, oat, coconut or almond milk (avoid almond for nut-free)

2 tsp lemon juice

240g/8½ oz/1¾ cups self-raising (self-rising) flour

200g/7 oz/1 cup caster (superfine) sugar

finely grated zest of 1 large lemon

100ml/3½ fl oz/scant ½ cup sunflower oil

½ tsp vanilla bean paste

3 tbsp freeze-dried raspberry pieces

In a large bowl, stir together the flour, sugar and lemon zest until combined. Whisk in the thickened milk as well as the oil, vanilla and freeze-dried raspberry pieces until you have a smooth loose batter.

Divide the batter between the muffin cases. I find this easier to do evenly with an ice-cream scoop although a jug or ladle are also good. The cases should be about two-thirds full.

Bake in the oven for 20 minutes until risen and golden. Turn the muffins out to cool on a wire rack.

For the frosting

200g/7 oz plant-based margarine or butter, softened

finely grated zest of 1 large lemon

400g/14 oz/3 cups icing (confectioners') sugar, sifted

freeze-dried raspberry pieces, to decorate

To make the frosting, beat together the margarine or butter and lemon zest until smooth. Add the icing sugar and beat well until light and creamy. If you want the frosting to be softer, add a little lemon juice.

Pipe or spread the frosting on top of the cooled cupcakes and finish with a sprinkling of freeze-dried raspberry pieces.

Flexible

*Flavour swap: to make **vanilla cupcakes**, swap the lemon juice for 2 teaspoons white wine vinegar or apple cider vinegar. Omit the lemon zest in the cake mix and double the amount of vanilla to 2 teaspoons. For the frosting, simply swap the lemon zest for 2 teaspoons vanilla bean paste.*

*To make **raspberry, rose and pistachio cupcakes**, swap the lemon juice for 2 teaspoons white wine vinegar or apple cider vinegar. Omit the lemon zest in the cake mix, then add in 50g / 1¾ oz finely chopped pistachios. For the frosting, swap the lemon zest for 1 teaspoon rosewater and a few drops of pink food colouring. Decorate the tops with freeze-dried raspberry pieces and more chopped pistachios.*

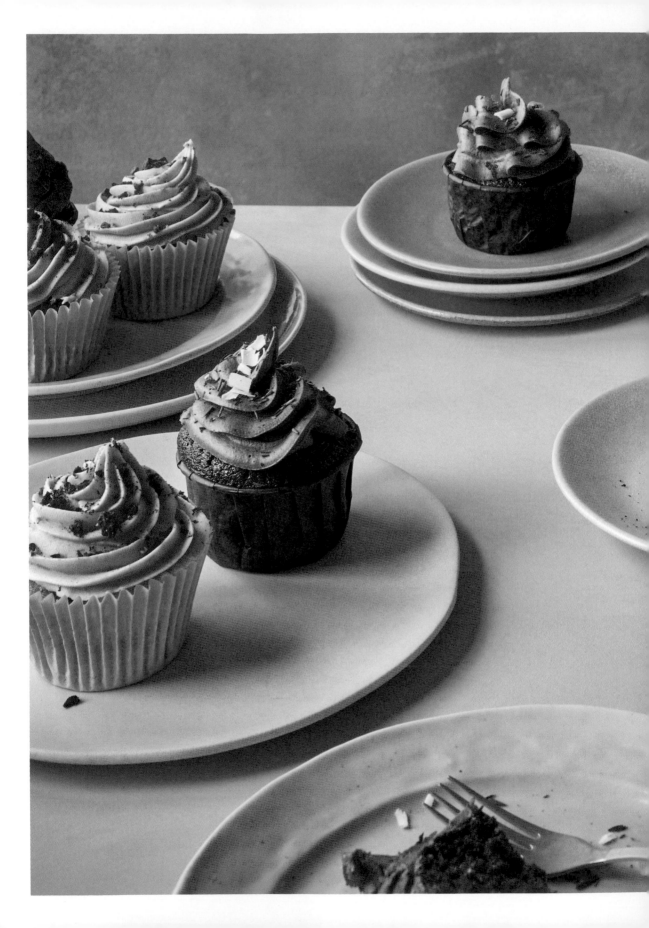

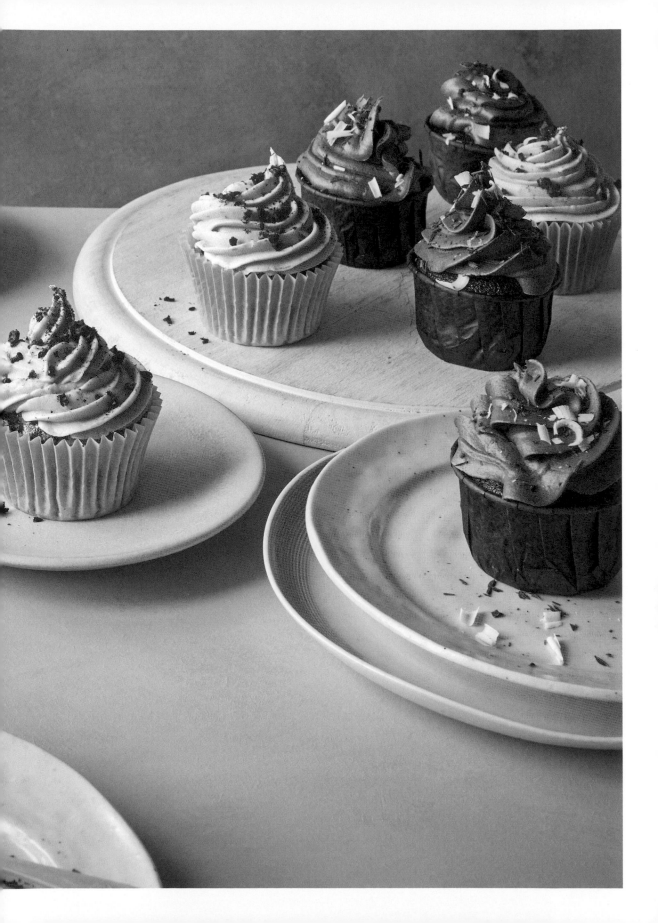

All-in-one chocolate fudge cake

This is based on a recipe my grandma and my mum always used to make when we had a birthday to celebrate. It's failsafe, super moist and lasts for days. The heavenly fudge frosting is silky smooth and stays that way once the cake is frosted, rather than setting over time. One tip I've learned for the lightest and smoothest end result, is to make sure your butter is really soft before making the frosting.

For the cake

250g/9 oz/1¾ cups plain (all-purpose)
  flour
75g/2¾ oz/¾ cup cocoa powder
1½ tsp bicarbonate of (baking) soda
1 tsp baking powder
150g/5½ oz/¾ cup caster (superfine)
  sugar
150g/5½ oz/¾ cup soft light brown sugar
225ml/8 fl oz/1 cup soured cream
225ml/8 fl oz/scant 1 cup black coffee, hot
2 eggs, beaten
100ml/3½ oz/scant ½ cup sunflower oil,
  plus extra for greasing
½ tsp fine sea salt

For the frosting

125g/4½ oz dark chocolate
  (70 per cent cocoa solids), chopped
225g/8 oz/1 cup butter, softened
40g/1½ oz golden (corn) syrup
75g/2¾ oz/½ cup icing (confectioners')
  sugar
40g/1½ oz/½ cup cocoa powder
100ml/3½ fl oz/½ cup soured cream
1 tsp vanilla bean paste
your choice of sprinkles, fudge pieces
  or grated chocolate, to decorate

Prep 40 minutes / **Cooking** 50 minutes–1 hour / **Serves** 10–12

Heat the oven to 180°C/160°C fan/350°F/gas 4 Brush a deep 20cm/ 8 inch cake tin with oil and line the base with baking parchment.

To make the cake, sift the flour, cocoa powder, bicarbonate of soda and baking powder into a large bowl and add the remaining ingredients. Whisk together until you have a loose smooth batter. Pour into the prepared tin and bake for 50 minutes–1 hour until the cake is springy to touch and starts to come away from the sides of the tin. To be sure the cake is cooked through, you can insert a skewer into the centre and it should come out clean. It's likely to rise more in the middle, which is fine as when you spread on the frosting this creates a domed effect.

Cool in the tin for 10 minutes before turning out and cooling completely on a wire rack.

To make the frosting, place the chocolate in a bowl over a pan of barely simmering water to slowly melt. Alternatively, gently melt in the microwave in 10-second bursts. Set aside to cool for 10 minutes.

Beat the butter on a high speed until it's really smooth and creamy. Add the golden syrup and sift in the icing sugar and cocoa powder. Beat for a few minutes until it's really light and fluffy. Add the soured cream, vanilla and cooled melted chocolate and beat on a low speed until smooth and silky.

Generously spread the frosting over the top and sides of the cake and decorate with sprinkles, fudge pieces or grated chocolate – or simply leave plain, if you like.

Flexible

Dairy-free: *swap the soured cream used in the cake and frosting for a plant-based natural yoghurt such as coconut or soya. Use a plant-based butter and dairy-free chocolate in the frosting. Alternatively, you could use the chocolate frosting from the chocolate cupcakes on page 78 to decorate this cake.*

Flavour swap: *for a malted chocolate cake, swap 25g / 1 oz cocoa powder for 25g / 1 oz malted milk powder.*

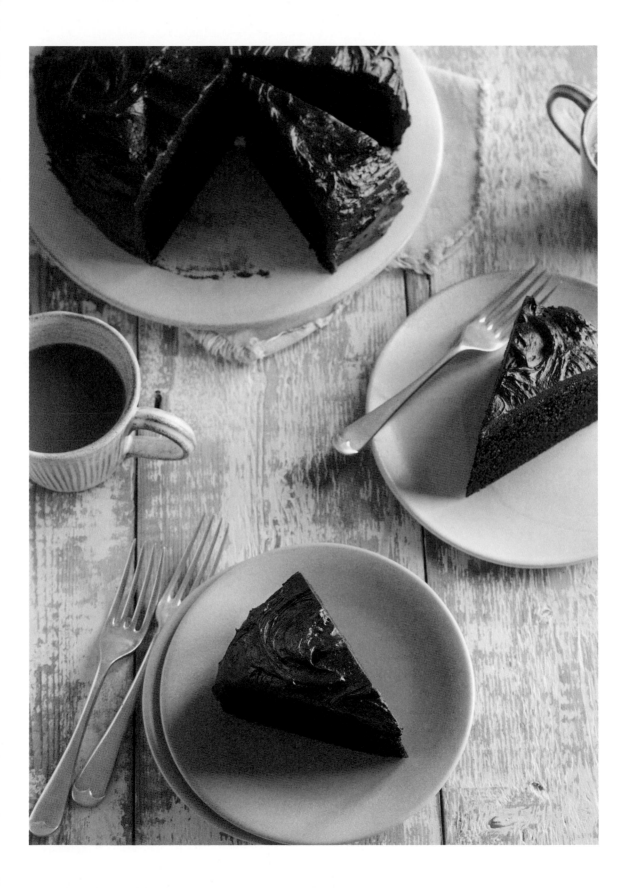

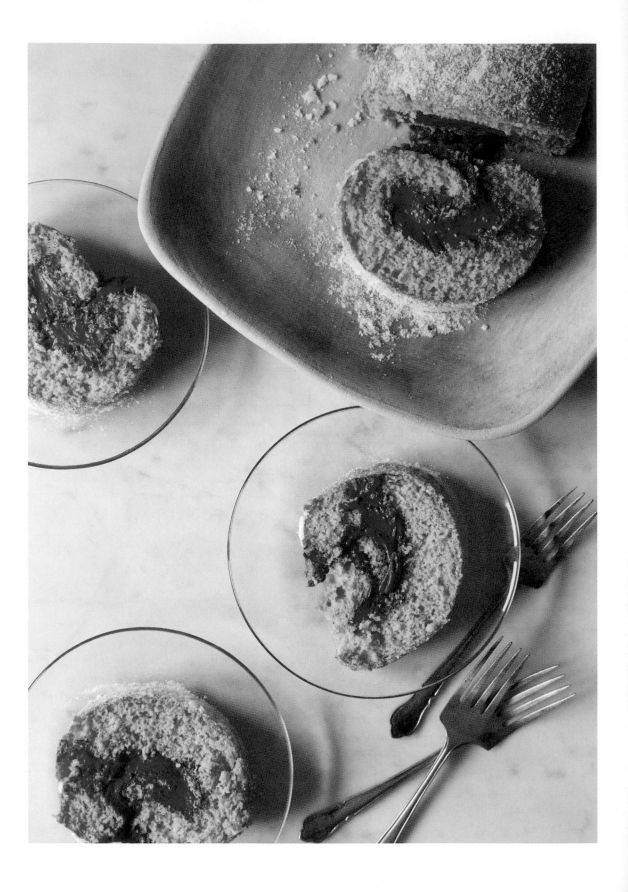

Blackcurrant and elderflower swiss roll

This whisked sponge is super light and incredibly soft. It's simple to make and amazingly uses just three ingredients. Classic Swiss roll recipes will have a fruit jam filling, but I wanted to make this into something a little more special with the tangy blackcurrant purée and lightly whipped elderflower-flavoured cream. The perfect summer cake.

For the Swiss roll

4 eggs

125g/4½ oz/⅔ cup caster (superfine) sugar, plus extra for dusting

125g/4½ oz/1 cup self-raising (self-rising) flour

sunflower oil, for greasing

For the filling

200g/7 oz/2 cups blackcurrants

50g/1¾ oz/¼ cup caster (superfine) sugar

200ml/7 fl oz/generous ¾ cup double (heavy) cream

2 tbsp elderflower cordial

Prep 40 minutes / **Cooking** 10–12 minutes / **Serves** 6–8

For the filling, put the blackcurrants in a small saucepan with the sugar and 3 tablespoons water. Bring to a simmer and cook for 5–7 minutes until the berries are completely soft. Blend to a purée and push through a sieve to remove any seeds. Leave to cool, then chill.

Heat the oven to 180°C/160°C fan/350°F/gas 4. Lightly brush the base of a Swiss roll tin with the oil. Line with baking parchment.

Using an electric mixer, whisk together the eggs and sugar for about 5 minutes until pale and creamy and doubled in volume. Sift half of the flour on top and gently fold in using a large metal spoon. Repeat with the remaining flour and fold in until there is no flour visible. Finish by folding in 1 tablespoon warm water, which helps give a lighter airy sponge when cooked.

Pour into the tin, lightly spreading into all of the corners. Bake for 10–12 minutes until lightly golden and springy to touch.

Cut a piece of baking parchment slightly bigger than the sponge and dust heavily with sugar. Carefully and swiftly turn the cooked sponge upside down onto the sugared surface and carefully peel away the lining parchment from the top. Cover with a clean tea towel to keep the sponge moist and leave it to cool completely.

Whisk together the cream and elderflower cordial until it starts to form peaks. Stir in the purée and spread over the cooled sponge, leaving a 2cm/¾ inch border. Starting at one long edge of the sponge, gently roll the sponge away from you into a log shape, ending with the seam underneath. Serve sprinkled with sugar.

Flexible

*Flavour swap: For a **Black Forest swiss roll** – cut the quantity of self-raising flour to 75g / 2¾ oz / ⅔ cup, and sieve together with 50g / 1¾ oz / ½ cup cocoa powder and ½ tsp baking powder. Make the sponge as above. For the filling, simply use 250g / 9oz good-quality black cherry jam or compote. Spread on top of the cooked chocolate sponge. Whisk the double cream with 2 tablespoons kirsch (cherry liqueur) and spread over the cherry layer. Roll up the swiss roll and decorate with some dark chocolate shavings.*

Festive almond, olive oil and orange cake

If you're not a fan of classic fruit cake-based Christmas cakes, or simply forget to make one in time for it to mature before the festive period, then this is a fantastic alternative. The cake can be served warm as a dessert, but as it's based on an oil and almond batter, it will stay moist for a few days and is equally as rewarding with a cup of tea in the afternoon.

For the cake
4 eggs
100g/3½ oz/½ cup caster (superfine)
   sugar
125ml/4 fl oz/½ cup olive oil, plus extra
   for greasing
finely grated zest of 1 orange,
   plus extra zest to decorate
4 tbsp orange juice
375g/13 oz/2¾ cups ground almonds
1 tsp baking powder (gluten-free)
½ tsp ground cinnamon
½ tsp ground ginger
½ tsp grated nutmeg
25g/1 oz flaked (slivered)
   almonds, toasted

For the syrup
100g/3½ oz honey
90ml/3 fl oz/⅓ cup orange juice
1 cinnamon stick
12 whole cloves

Prep 25 minutess / **Cooking** 45 minutes / **Serves** 10–12

Heat the oven to 160°C/140°C fan/325°F/gas 3. Brush a 22cm/8½ inch loose-bottomed or springform cake tin with oil and line the base with baking parchment.

To make the cake, put the eggs and sugar in a large bowl and whisk for around 5 minutes or until very light and fluffy. Add the olive oil, orange zest and juice and briefly mix in before adding the ground almonds, baking powder and ground spices. Stir to combine and transfer to the prepared cake tin. Bake in the oven for 45 minutes until risen, golden and just firm to touch.

While the cake is cooking, make the syrup. Put the honey, orange juice, cinnamon stick and cloves in a small saucepan and place over a medium heat. Bring to the boil and cook for about 5 minutes or until it is thickened, reduced by half and syrupy.

Cool the cake in the tin for 10 minutes before removing and placing on a serving plate. Remove the whole spices from the syrup if preferred, and pour over the warm cake. Finish by scattering over the flaked almonds, grate over some orange zest and serve warm.

Flexible

Nut-free: you can swap the ground almonds for desiccated (shredded) coconut, although it's best to blitz the coconut briefly in a food processor first to give it a finer consistency. Finish the cake with toasted coconut flakes on top.

*Flavour swap: to make this into a **lemon and rosemary cake**, swap the orange juice and zest in the cake for lemon zest and juice. Omit the dried spices. For the syrup, use 100ml / 3½ fl oz / scant ½ cup lemon juice with 100g / 3½ oz honey, and swap the cinnamon and cloves for 2 stalks of rosemary that have been bashed with a rolling pin to extract flavour.*

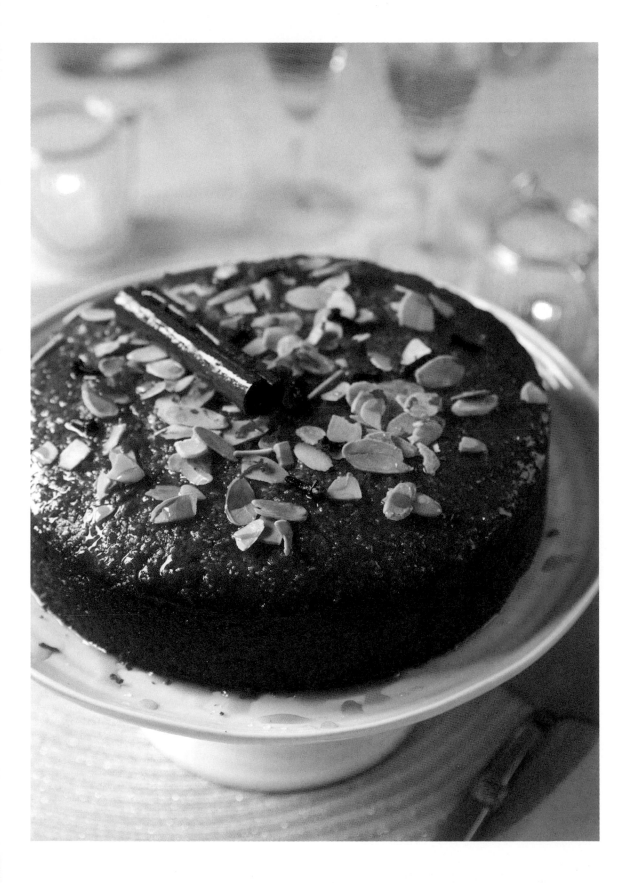

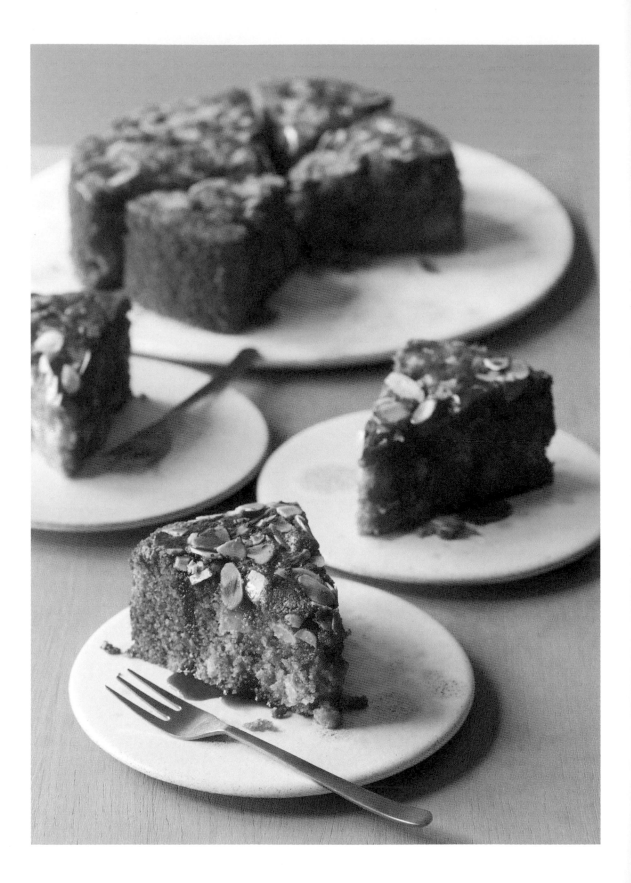

Apple and cinnamon polenta cake

with maple syrup

I'd say this is the best cake to serve for anyone who favours savoury over sweet, like Olly my son. He's not one for desserts but this cake he'll ask for more of every time it's made. I think it's the tartness from the apple, warmth from the cinnamon and slight crunch of polenta.

Polenta cakes are very robust and work well when mixed with fresh fruits. As the fruit cooks and releases juices, these are soaked up by the polenta, giving a light-textured cake rather than a heavy one. This gluten-free cake would be just as lovely served as a mid-morning or afternoon treat, as well as a dessert or even with a glass of milk before bed (yes Olly, I've seen you!).

200g/7 oz/¾ cup butter, softened

200g/7 oz/1 cup caster (superfine) sugar

3 eggs

200g/7 oz/2 cups ground almonds

100g/3½ oz/⅔ cup polenta (cornmeal)

2 tbsp cornflour (cornstarch)

1½ tsp baking powder

1 tsp ground cinnamon

200g/7 oz cooking apple, peeled and cored

20g/¾ oz flaked (slivered) almonds

100ml/3½ fl oz/scant ½ cup maple syrup

Prep 25 minutes / **Cooking** 45 minutes / **Serves** 8–10

Heat the oven to 180°C/160°C fan/350°F/gas 4. Grease and line a 23cm/9 inch loose-bottomed or springform cake tin with baking parchment.

In a large bowl, beat together the butter and sugar with an electric whisk for 2 minutes or until light and fluffy. Add the eggs, one at a time, mixing well between additions.

Mix together the ground almonds, polenta, cornflour, baking powder and cinnamon in a separate bowl and mix well. Lightly fold the dry mixture into the butter, sugar and egg mixture until just smooth.

Cut the apple into small chunks, no bigger than 1cm/½ inch big. Fold through the cake batter and spoon into the prepared tin. Scatter over the flaked almonds and bake for 45 minutes until golden and a skewer inserted into the centre comes out clean.

As soon as the cake comes out, drizzle the maple syrup all over the top and leave to soak in for 10 minutes before transferring to a wire rack to cool completely before serving.

Flexible

Nut-free: *desiccated (shredded) coconut is a great alternative to the ground almonds, however, you are best to blitz them to a finer texture in a food processor before using. You can also swap the flaked (slivered) almonds for some coconut flakes.*

Flavour swap: *to make this into an **orange and raspberry cake**, swap the ground cinnamon with the finely grated zest of 1 orange and use 200g / 7 oz / 1⅔ cups raspberries instead of the apple. As an alternative to drizzling with maple syrup once cooked, make a syrup by boiling the juice of the zested orange with 3 tablespoons caster (superfine) sugar for around 1 minute until syrupy and pour over the cooked cake.*

Espresso and walnut cake

There is something about these two flavours that work so well together. However, they can often be a little bland, so here I've made them both really shout out. Strong espresso coffee is in both the cake and the cream cheese frosting. As for the walnuts, they are blitzed into the cake batter, which also contains some walnut oil. Then the walnuts on top are made extra special by caramelising in sugar.

For the cake

300g/10½ oz/1½ cups soft light brown sugar

75g/2¾ oz/½ cup walnut pieces

325g/11½ oz/2½ cups plain (all-purpose) flour

1 tsp baking powder

1½ tsp bicarbonate of (baking) soda

2 eggs

225ml/8 fl oz/1 cup soured cream

100ml/3½ fl oz/scant ½ cup walnut oil

4 tbsp instant espresso powder, dissolved in 175ml/6 fl oz/¾ cup hot water

½ tsp ground cinnamon

½ tsp fine sea salt

For the frosting

75g/2¾ oz/⅓ cup butter, softened

125g/4½ oz/½ cup cream cheese

300g/10½ oz/2 cups icing (confectioners') sugar, sifted

½ tsp ground cinnamon

1 tbsp instant espresso powder, dissolved in 1 tbsp hot water

To decorate

75g/2¾ oz/⅓ cup caster (superfine) sugar

75g/2¾ oz/½ cup walnut pieces

Prep 30 minutes / **Cooking** 30 minutes / **Serves** 12

Heat the oven to 180°C/160°C fan/350°F/gas 4. Oil and line two 20cm/8 inch cake tins with baking parchment.

To make the cake, put the sugar and walnuts in a food processor and blitz to finely chop the walnuts. Add all of the remaining cake ingredients, and blitz well to give you a smooth, loose batter. Divide the cake mix between the two tins.

Bake for 25–30 minutes until the cakes are risen and springy to touch and start to come away from the sides of the tins. Cool in the tins for 10 minutes before removing and cooling completely on a wire rack.

While the cake is cooling, make the frosting. Beat the butter in an electric mixer until smooth. Add the cream cheese, beating for about a minute until smooth. Reduce the speed to low, then add the icing sugar, cinnamon and espresso. Beat until you have a smooth and creamy texture.

Spread half of the frosting on top of one of the cakes and sandwich the other on top. Spread the remaining frosting on top.

To prepare the decoration, line a baking tray with baking parchment. Put the sugar in a small saucepan over a medium heat and leave until the sugar is melted and deep golden, swirling the pan a couple of times for even colour. Don't leave the pan unattended, as it can burn very quickly. Immediately tip the walnuts into the pan, stir to coat in the caramel and tip onto the prepared tray, flattening into a single layer with the spoon. The nuts will become cold and crunchy. You can either leave them in large pieces to decorate the top of the cake, or crush them into smaller pieces with a rolling pin and sprinkle over the cake.

Flexible

Gluten-free: *a gluten-free flour blend will work very well in this cake.*

Flavour swap: *to make a **mocha and pecan cake**, replace 60g/ 2 oz/scant ½ cup of the flour with 60g/2 oz/generous ½ cup cocoa powder and use pecan nuts instead of walnuts in both the cake and the decoration. Replace the walnut oil with sunflower oil.*

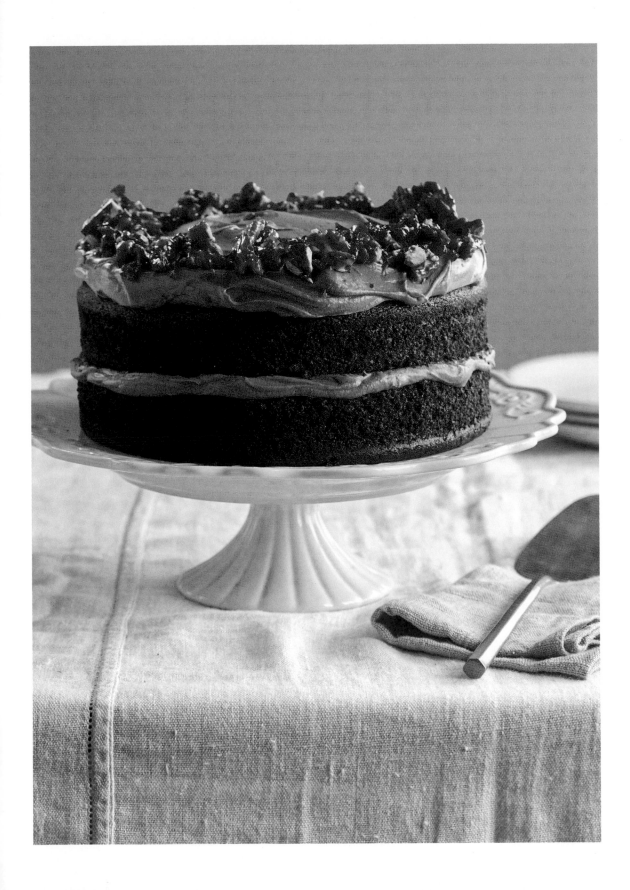

Brown butter honey buns

*These are a cross between a spiced
Scandinavian honey cake and the
classic hot cross bun with their warm
spices and dried fruit. These may
look like a muffin, but they have a
drier texture that seems to get better
over a couple of days. Enjoy as they
are, lightly warmed through, or serve
split in half, toasted and spread with
salted butter. As an alternative serving
suggestion, try the honey cream cheese
frosting in the Flexible section below.*

150g/5½ oz/⅔ cup butter

100g/3½ oz honey

100g/3½ oz/½ cup soft light brown sugar

½ tsp flaked sea salt

200g/7 oz/1½ cups plain (all-purpose)
  flour

1½ tsp bicarbonate of (baking) soda

1 tsp ground mixed (apple pie) spice

100g/3½ oz/⅔ cup sultanas (golden
  raisins)

3 eggs, beaten

Prep 25 minutes / **Cooking** 20 minutes / **Makes** 10

Put the butter in a small saucepan over a medium heat, stirring
frequently. The butter will melt and splatter, then start to foam.
Once you start to see dark golden flecks, remove the pan from the
heat. Add the honey, sugar and salt, stirring until the sugar has
dissolved. Set aside to cool for 10 minutes.

Heat the oven to 180°C/160°C fan/350°F/gas 4. Line a deep muffin
tin with 10 muffin cases.

Put the flour, bicarbonate of soda, mixed spice and sultanas in a
bowl and stir together. Make a well in the centre and add the eggs
and cooled brown butter honey mixture. Mix everything together to
make a batter.

Divide the batter between the muffin cases and bake for 20 minutes
until they are risen and golden, and a skewer comes out clean when
inserted in the middle. Turn the muffins out to cool on a wire rack.
Serve warm with salted butter or lightly toasted as described above.

Flexible

Flavour swap: *for a fruitier flavour, 100g / 3½ oz / ⅔ cup
candied mixed peel is delicious instead of the sultanas
(golden raisins), or a mixture of the two is also very good.*

*For **honey cream cheese frosting**, beat together 150g /
5½ oz / ¾ cup cream cheese, 50g / 1¾ oz / softened butter and
5 tablespoons honey. Spread on top of the buns once cool.*

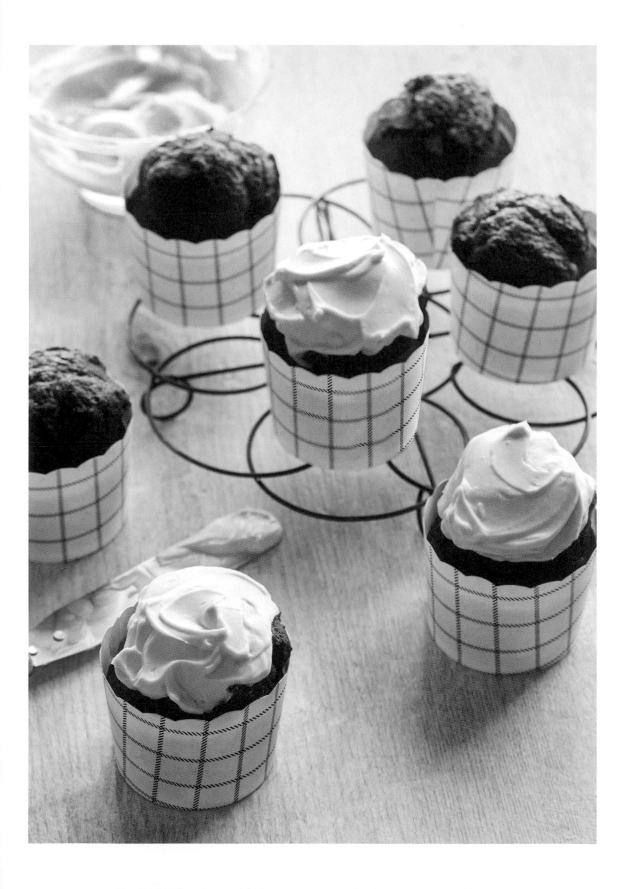

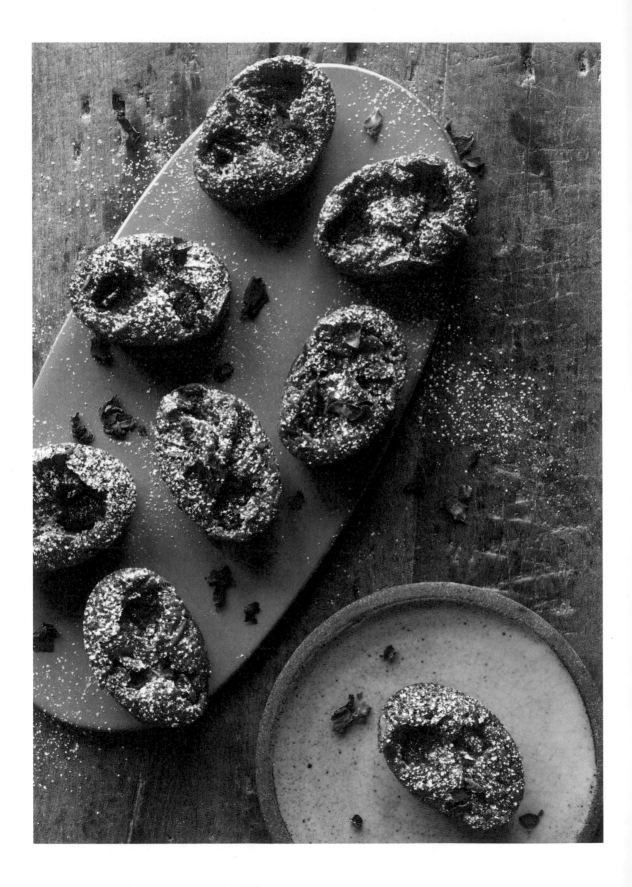

Raspberry, pistachio and rose friands

Friands are small, oval-shaped cakes originating in France that are made using ground nuts and egg whites, giving them a light texture. They can be flavoured with fruit, spices, chocolate or citrus zests. These friands are delicately flavoured with ground pistachios, raspberries and rosewater. If you can't get hold of a friand mould, you can just as easily bake them in a muffin tin. Please do make sure you use frozen raspberries for this recipe as they retain their shape far better and make a lighter friand sponge when cooked.

125g/4½ oz/½ cup butter, plus extra for greasing

125g/4½ oz pistachio nuts

150g/5½ oz/1 cup icing (confectioners') sugar, plus extra for dusting

50g/1½ oz/½ cup cornflour (cornstarch)

3 egg whites

½ tsp rosewater

100g/3½ oz/1 cup frozen raspberries

dried rose petals, to serve (optional)

Prep 25 minutes / **Cooking** 30 minutes / **Makes** 8

Heat the oven to 180°C/160°C fan/350°F/gas 4. Grease 8 friand moulds or if you don't have friand moulds use a non-stick muffin tin or mini loaf cases.

Melt the butter and set aside to cool slightly.

Roughly chop 25g/1 oz of the pistachio nuts and set aside. Put the remaining 100g/3½ oz in a food processor and blitz until they are finely ground. Add the icing sugar and cornflour. Blitz to combine, then transfer to a large mixing bowl

In a separate bowl, whisk the egg whites until they become a soft foam consistency. Make a well in the dry ingredients and pour in the egg whites along with the cooled melted butter and rosewater. Gently mix to give you a soft batter.

Divide the mixture between the moulds – I find using an ice-cream scoop works well for this. Sit a few frozen raspberries on top of each one and scatter over the reserved chopped pistachios. Bake for 25–30 minutes until they are lightly golden and firm.

Cool in the mould for a few minutes before carefully turning out onto a wire rack to cool to room temperature.

Serve scattered with dried rose petals, if using, and dusted with icing sugar.

Flexible

Nut-free: *desiccated (shredded) coconut is a great alternative to the pistachio nuts. Blitz the coconut in a food processor to create a finer texture before using.*

Flavour swap: *to make **lemon and blueberry friands**, swap the rosewater for the finely grated zest of 1 lemon and use blueberries instead of raspberries.*

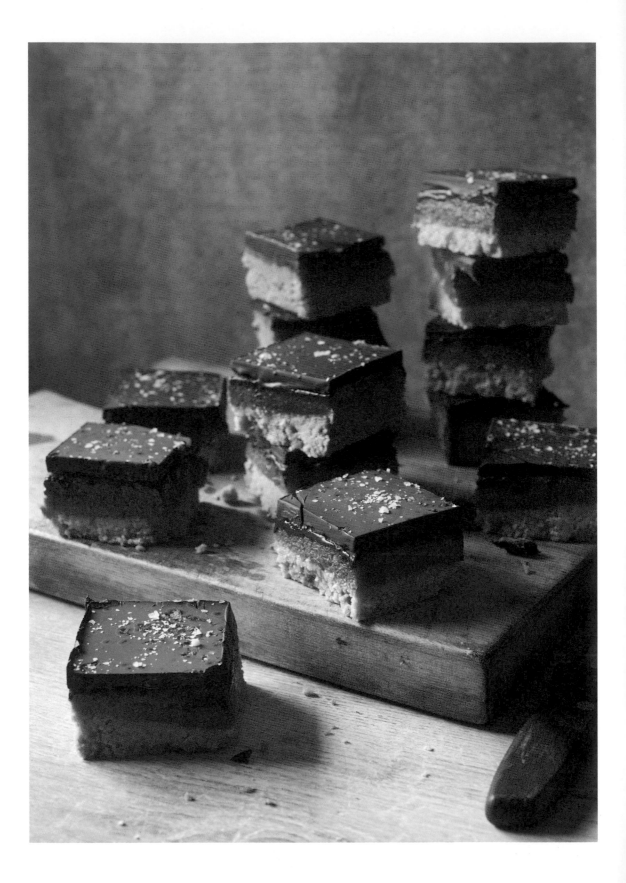

Multi-millionaire's shortbread

What gives these their multi-millionaire status I hear you ask? It's mainly about the shortbread. I actually use a gluten-free flour blend as it stays crisp and light compared to a wheat flour, which can be a little doughy. Rather than using plain butter, I have caramelised it first for added depth of flavour. To top things off, I add a good sprinkling of flaked sea salt into the caramel for total deliciousness.

For the shortbread

250g/9 oz/1 cup butter, plus extra for
   greasing
300g/10½ oz/2¼ cups gluten-free flour
100g/3½ oz/½ cup caster (superfine)
   sugar
¼ tsp flaked sea salt

For the caramel

397g/14 oz can condensed milk
150g/5½ oz/⅔ cup butter
150g/5½ oz/¾ cup caster (superfine)
   sugar
75g/2¾ oz golden (corn) syrup
½ tsp flaked sea salt

For the topping

250g/9 oz dark chocolate (70 per cent
   cocoa solids), chopped
½ tsp flaked sea salt

Prep 35 minutes, plus 1¼ hours chilling / **Cooking** 25 minutes / **Makes** 20 small (but very rich) pieces

To make the brown butter shortbread, put the butter in a saucepan over a medium heat, stirring frequently. Once you start to see dark golden flecks, remove the pan from the heat. Transfer to a heatproof bowl, then chill in the fridge until set.

Heat the oven to 180°C/160°C fan/350°F/gas 4. Grease and line the base of a 20cm/8 inch square tin.

Remove the set brown butter from the fridge. Put into a food processor with the flour, sugar and salt. Blitz until it is crumbly. Tip into the prepared tin and push down with the back of a spoon until you have an even base. Bake for 20–25 minutes until lightly golden, soft and bubbling. Leave to cool and set firm in the tin.

For the caramel, put all of the ingredients in a heavy-based saucepan and place over a low heat. Stir continuously for 10 minutes, or until the caramel has started to thicken and becomes a golden colour. Pour over the shortbread. Set aside to cool for about 30 minutes.

Finally, make the topping. Place the chocolate in a bowl over a pan of barely simmering water to melt. Alternatively, melt in the microwave in 10-second bursts. Pour this over the salted caramel layer (the caramel doesn't have to be totally set). Sprinkle over the salt, then chill in the fridge for the chocolate to set.

After about 30 minutes, carefully remove from the tin and cut into small squares with a sharp knife.

Flexible

Vegan: to make the shortbread base (this won't be a brown butter base), blend together 200g / 7 oz plant-based butter, 300g / 10½ oz / 2¼ cups gluten-free flour, 100g / 3½ oz / ½ cup caster (superfine) sugar and ½ teaspoon flaked sea salt until you have a crumbly texture. Press into the tin and bake as above. For the caramel, use a vegan condensed milk and plant-based butter, making the caramel in the same way as the above recipe, with the addition of 1 tablespoon cornflour (cornstarch) mixed in. Finally, make sure you use a dairy-free dark chocolate to melt and pour over the top.

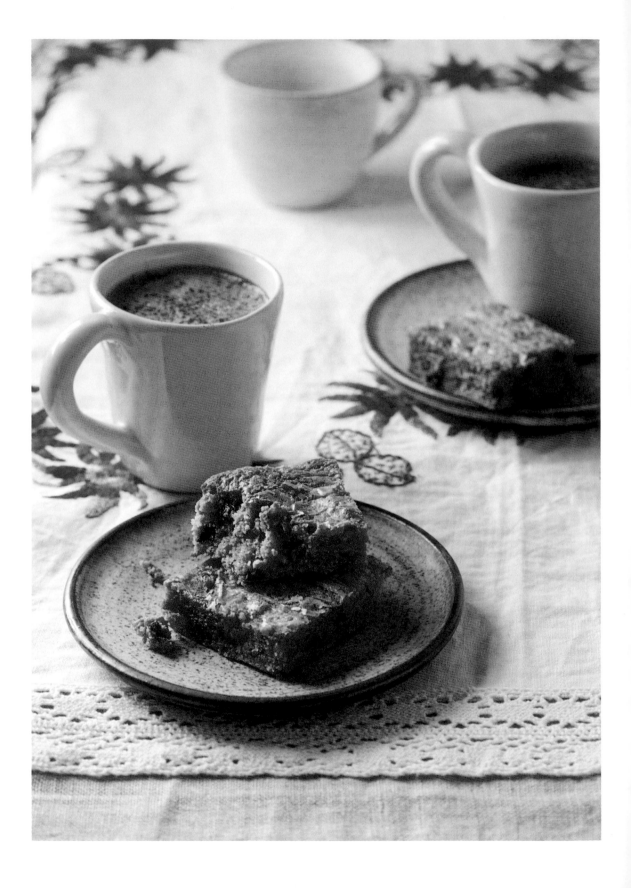

White chocolate and tahini blondies

These are rather naughty but very nice indeed. The addition of tahini in the vanilla and white chocolate blondie cuts through the sweetness, giving them a mellow sesame flavour. Though don't get me wrong – these are definitely for those with a sweet tooth.

Once made, they'll last for up to a week and still maintain a lovely texture, though it's highly unlikely they'll hang around for that long!

200g/7 oz/¾ cup butter, plus extra
    for greasing
200g/7 oz white chocolate, chopped
3 eggs
175g/6 oz/scant 1 cup soft light brown
    sugar
2 tsp vanilla bean paste
125g/4½ oz tahini
125g/4½ oz/1 cup plain (all-purpose) flour
½ tsp fine sea salt
100g/3½ oz milk or dark chocolate
    chunks, or toasted hazelnuts,
    roughly chopped

Prep 35 minutes, plus 1 hour cooling / **Cooking** 25 minutes / **Makes** 15 squares

Heat the oven to 180°C/160°C fan/350°F/gas 4. Grease and line a 20 x 30cm/8 x 12 inch rectangular, 4cm/1½ inch deep baking tin with baking parchment.

Place the butter and white chocolate in a bowl over a pan of barely simmering water to slowly melt. Alternatively, gently melt in the microwave in 10-second bursts.

In a separate large bowl, whisk together the eggs, sugar and vanilla until they are thick and creamy.

Stir the tahini into the chocolate and butter and pour into the egg mixture. Whisk well until combined. Add the flour and salt, stirring until all of the flour is mixed in. Fold through the chocolate chunks or hazelnuts.

Pour into the baking tin and bake for 25 minutes until the top is cracking and the centre is just set. Leave to cool in the tin for at least 1 hour before cutting into squares.

Flexible

__Gluten-free:__ gluten-free plain (all-purpose) flour works well as a direct swap for the plain (all-purpose) flour. However, for a delicate coconut flavour in the blondies, coconut flour is really delicious.

*__Flavour swap:__ to make **peanut butter blondies** simply swap the tahini for a smooth peanut butter and stir through 100g / 3½ oz roughly chopped unsalted roasted peanuts into the batter before baking.*

Double choc chip brookies

Could things get any better – delicious chocolate chip cookie base, topped with rich gooey brownie batter, all baked to perfection? The cookie layer is made using olive oil, which makes them slightly crispy, stopping them from becoming too doughy, and the brownies just melt in your mouth. Whip together a tray of these beauties and you'll be everyone's favourite friend. They are utter indulgence.

For the base

300g/10½ oz/2¼ cups plain (all-purpose) flour

1 tsp baking powder

1 tsp bicarbonate of (baking) soda

200g/7 oz milk or dark chocolate chips

½ tsp fine sea salt

150ml/5 fl oz olive oil

175g/2¾ oz/scant 1 cup soft light brown sugar

1 tsp vanilla bean paste

For the topping

125g/4½ oz/½ cup butter

125g/4½ oz dark chocolate (70 per cent cocoa solids), chopped

2 eggs

200g/7 oz/1 cup caster (superfine) sugar

1 tsp vanilla bean paste

85g/3 oz/⅔ cup plain (all-purpose) flour

¼ tsp fine sea salt

Prep 35 minutes / **Cooking** 25 minutes / **Makes** 20 squares

Heat the oven to 180°C/160°C fan/350°F/gas 4. Line a 20 x 30cm/ 8 x 12 inch rectangular, 4cm/1½ inch deep baking tin with baking parchment.

To make the cookie base, put the flour, baking powder, bicarbonate of soda, chocolate chips and salt in a large mixing bowl and stir to mix.

Mix together the oil, 75ml/2½ fl oz/⅓ cup water, the sugar and vanilla until combined and pour this into the flour. Stir until the dough just comes together without overmixing. Press loosely into the base of the prepared tin.

For the brownie layer, put the butter and chocolate in a bowl over a pan of barely simmering water to slowly melt. Alternatively, gently melt in the microwave in 10-second bursts.

In a separate bowl, whisk together the eggs, sugar and vanilla until they are thick and creamy. Pour in the melted chocolate and butter, and mix together.

Stir in the flour and salt, then pour on top of the cookie base and level the surface by giving the pan a gentle shake. Bake for about 25 minutes until the top is cracking and the centre is just set. Leave to cool in the tin for about 30 minutes before cutting into squares.

Flexible

Dairy-free: choose a suitable dairy-free chocolate and substitute the butter with a plant-based butter, or a light oil such as rapeseed (canola) or sunflower oil in the brownie batter. The results are a little softer and gooier but what's not to like about that!

Flavour swap: play around with flavours in the brownie batter such as the addition of: 1 teaspoon ground cinnamon or ginger, 1 tablespoon instant coffee powder dissolved in 1 tablespoon hot water or finely grated zest of 1 orange.

Or you could also add up to 250g / 9 oz of your choice of treat:

- *chocolate chips*

- *dried fruit*

- *mini marshmallows (just a couple of handfuls of these)*

- *chopped stem ginger or candied peel*

- *roughly chopped nuts*

- *fudge or caramel chunks*

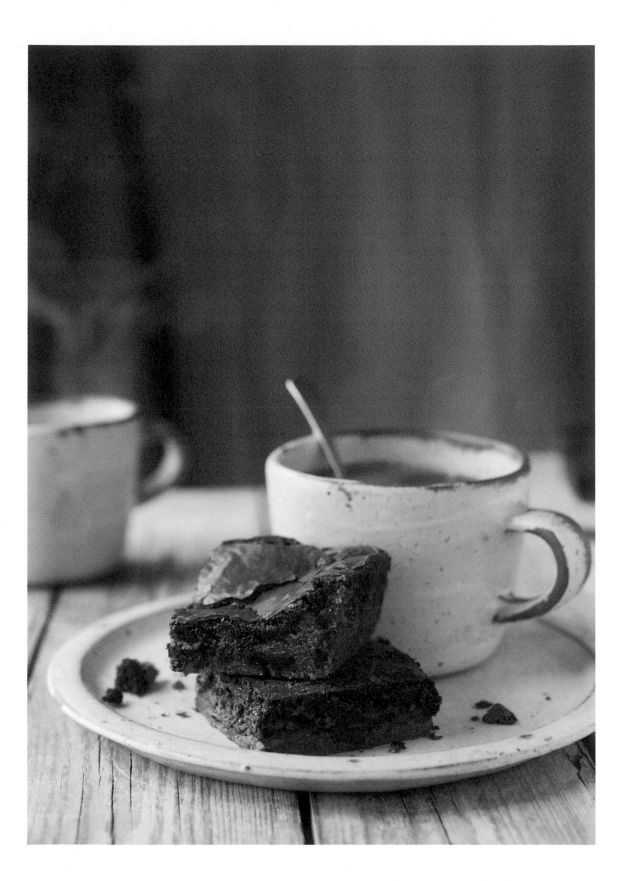

Rhubarb and ginger streusel traybake

This irresistible traybake has just the right balance of softness from the polenta sponge cake base, tartness from the chunks of juicy rhubarb, bites of ginger throughout and sweet crunch from the topping. Tuck into a piece with a morning coffee, afternoon cuppa, dessert with a dollop of soured cream or packed in a lunch box.

For the filling
650/1 lb 4 oz rhubarb, trimmed and
   cut into 2.5cm/1 inch pieces
60g/2 oz/generous ¼ cup caster
   (superfine) sugar
finely grated zest of ½ orange

For the topping
125g/4½ oz/scant 1 cup porridge
   (oatmeal) oats (gluten-free)
100g/3½ oz/1 cup ground almonds
100g/3½ oz/½ cup butter, diced
50g/1¾ oz/¼ cup caster (superfine) sugar
1 tsp ground ginger

For the base
175g/6 oz/¾ cup butter, softened, plus
   extra for greasing
200g/8 oz/1 cup caster (superfine) sugar
5 eggs
100g/3½ oz/1 cup ground almonds
100g/3½ oz/⅔ cup polenta (cornmeal)
1 tsp baking powder (gluten-free)
¼ tsp fine seal salt
75g/2¾ oz stem ginger, finely chopped

Prep 40 minutes, plus 30 minutes cooling / **Cooking** 50 minutes / **Makes** 20 squares

Heat the oven to 180°C/160°C fan/350°F/gas 4. Lightly grease a 23 x 30cm/9 x 12 inch deep baking tin and line the base with baking parchment.

For the filling, toss the rhubarb in the sugar and orange zest, and tip onto a baking tray. Bake for 15 minutes until it's tender and a little juicy. Set aside to cool while you make the other layers.

To make the streusel topping, put all the ingredients in a food processor and briefly blitz to give you a breadcrumb consistency.

For the base, using an electric mixer, beat together the butter and sugar for a few minutes until it is light and fluffy. Beat in the eggs one at a time, then beat in the ground almonds, polenta, baking powder, salt and ginger. Spread the batter into the prepared tin and spoon over the rhubarb in an even layer on top.

Scatter over the streusel topping and bake for 50 minutes until golden and the centre feels firm when lightly pressed. Cool in the tin for about 30 minutes before serving warm or turning out to cool completely on a wire rack.

Flexible

*Flavour swap: for a **blackberry and lemon streusel traybake**, omit the ground ginger in the streusel topping, swap the diced stem ginger for the grated zest of 2 lemons in the cake base, and use 400g/14 oz/3 cups fresh or frozen blackberries instead of the rhubarb, which can be scattered straight into the cake batter.*

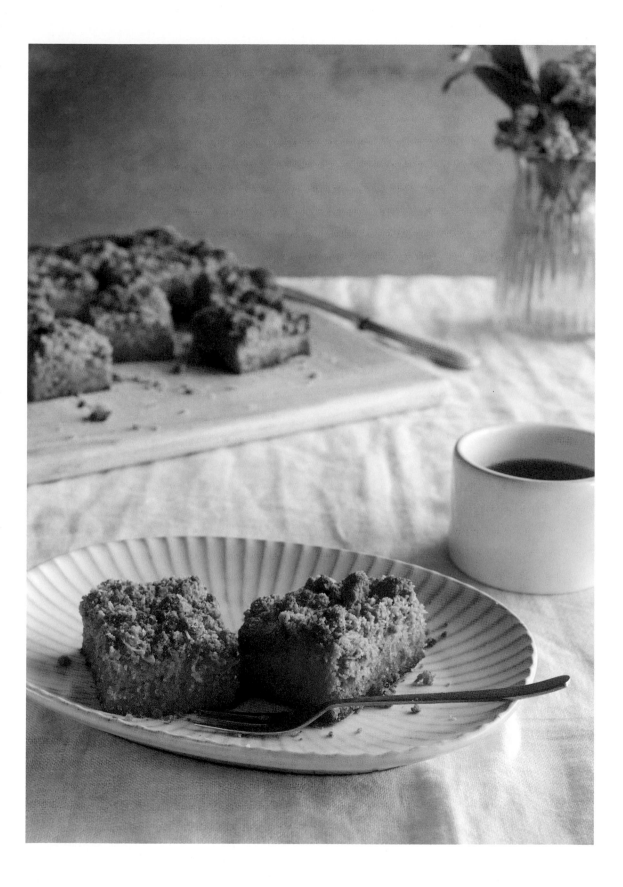

Banana caramel traybake

with caramel frosting

This banana traybake would be wonderful just on its own, but I wanted to make something even more special, so I've added a light and creamy caramel frosting. And if that's not enough, there is a generous drizzle of more caramel on top. As one friend put it when she first tried this, it is banana cake taken to a level beyond words.

For the cake

375g/13 oz/2¾ cups plain (all-purpose) flour

½ tsp fine sea salt

1½ tsp baking powder

½ tsp bicarbonate of (baking) soda

3 ripe bananas, mashed

175ml/6 fl oz/¾ cup natural yoghurt or buttermilk

150g/5½ oz/⅔ cup butter, softened, plus extra for greasing

100g/3½ oz/½ cup soft light brown sugar

100g/3½ oz/½ cup caster (superfine) sugar

2 tsp vanilla bean paste

2 eggs

60g/2 oz shop-bought caramel sauce

For the frosting

115g/4 oz/½ cup butter, softened

225g/8 oz/1⅔ cups icing (confectioners') sugar, sifted

50g/1¾ oz caramel sauce, plus extra to drizzle

Prep 35 minutes / **Cooking** 25 minutes / **Makes** 12–15 slices

Heat the oven to 180°C/160°C fan/350°F/gas 4. Lightly grease a 23 x 30cm/9 x 12 inch deep baking tin and line the base with a piece of baking parchment.

For the cake, mix together the flour, salt, baking powder and bicarbonate of soda. In a separate bowl, mix together the banana and yoghurt or buttermilk and set these aside.

In a large bowl, using an electric mixer, beat together the butter, sugars and vanilla until really light and creamy. Beat in the eggs, then add the flour mixture and banana mixture in 2 or 3 stages, alternating between each one and mixing gently between each addition to avoid overmixing. Once everything is just combined, spoon into the prepared tin. Drizzle over the caramel sauce (warming it a little if it is too thick to drizzle) and swirl into the batter, levelling off the surface with a spatula. Bake for 25–28 minutes, until golden and the centre feels just firm. A skewer should come out clean when inserted in the middle.

Let the cake cool completely in the tin before transferring to a board or large plate.

To make the frosting, beat together the butter and icing sugar for a couple of minutes until light and creamy, before beating in the caramel. Spread on top of the cake and finish with more caramel sauce drizzled on top.

Flexible

Vegan: use a plant-based butter and caramel sauce for the cake and frosting. As a replacement for the eggs, mix together 2 tablespoons ground flaxseed with 6 tablespoons cold water and leave to thicken for 10 minutes before using as you would the eggs. To replace the yoghurt or buttermilk, stir 1 tablespoon lemon juice into 175ml / 6 fl oz / ¾ cup plant-based milk, sit for a few minutes to thicken slightly and use as above.

Gluten-free: a gluten-free flour blend works just as well for this recipe, plus you will need to make sure the baking powder is gluten-free.

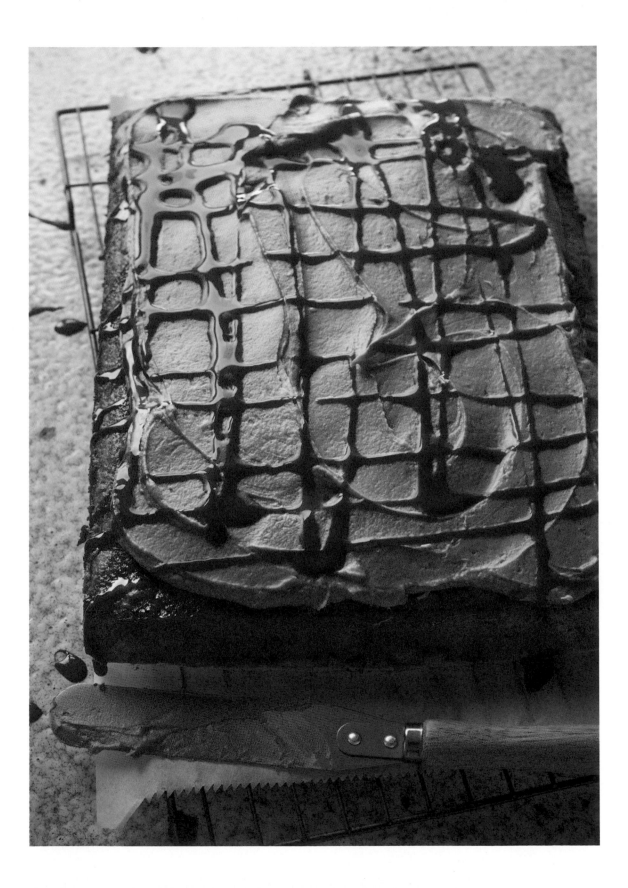

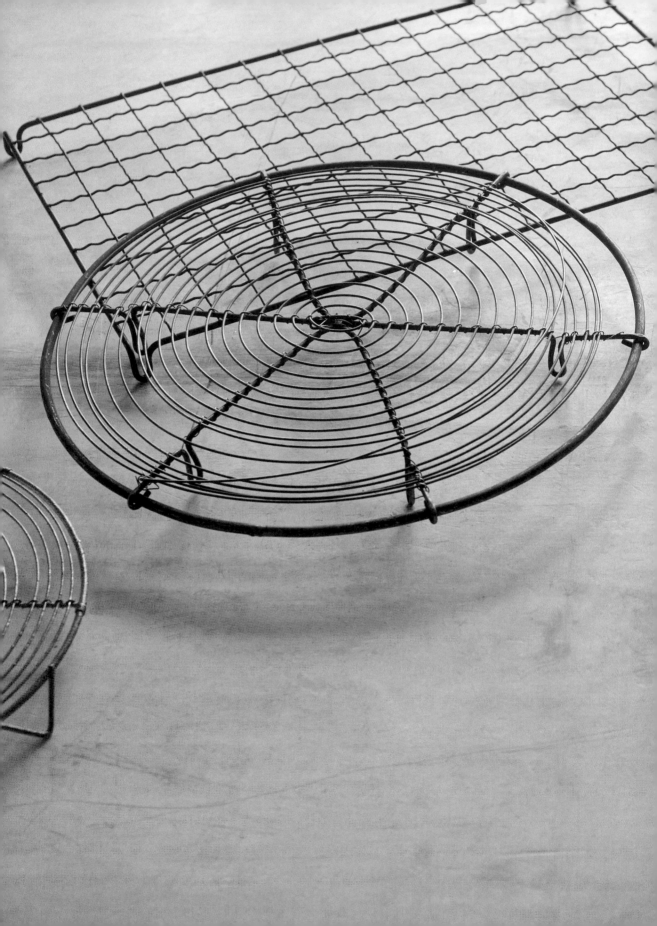

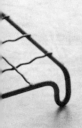

biscuits
and cookies

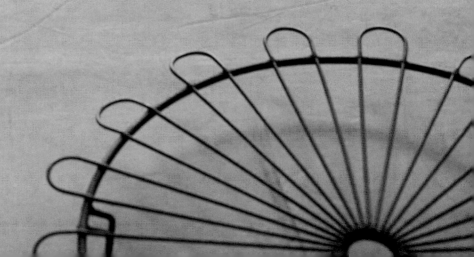

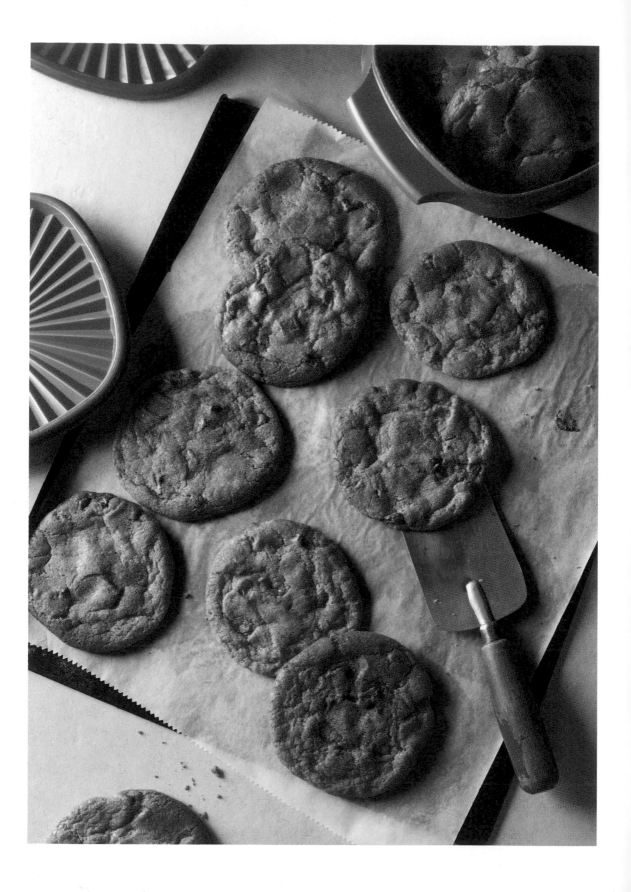

Rosa's chocolate orange cookies

I had to include these in this book, as out of all the baking that's done in my house these are probably made the most. My daughter Rosa has perfected the recipe over time and can now pretty much make them with her eyes closed. They have that perfect soft chewy texture and rich buttery flavour a cookie should have and can easily be customised with your favourite treat.

_____

125g/4½ oz/½ cup butter, softened
115g/4 oz/generous ½ cup soft light brown sugar
115g/4 oz/generous ½ cup caster (superfine) sugar
finely grated zest of ¼ orange
1 egg, beaten
1 tsp vanilla bean paste
225g/8 oz/1¾ cups self-raising (self-rising) flour
½ tsp flaked sea salt
200g/7 oz milk chocolate chunks

Prep 15 minutes / **Cooking** 7–9 minutes / **Makes** 16

Heat the oven to 200°C/180°C fan/400°F/gas 6. Line two baking trays with baking parchment.

In a large bowl, beat together the butter, sugars and orange zest until light and creamy. Add the egg and vanilla, beating until combined.

Mix in the flour, salt and chocolate chunks until you have a dough.

Roll into 16 walnut-size balls and put on the baking tray spaced well apart to allow for spreading, baking in batches if necessary.

Bake for 7 minutes for a soft-baked cookie or leaving a couple of extra minutes for a firmer crunch. Cool for a few minutes on the trays before transferring to wire racks to cool.

Flexible

Flavour swap: *as an alternative to the chocolate chunks in the recipe you can add your favourite chocolate treats into the cookie dough instead: 200g/7 oz Smarties, M&M's, chocolate orange, white chocolate, dark chocolate or caramel bar broken into chunks, Maltesers, mini marshmallows (just a couple of handfuls), toffee pieces all work well.*

Giant chocolate and peanut butter sharing cookie

This huge cookie is perfect for sharing, whether it's for a bunch of teenagers who descend upon your house after school and are likely to eat you out of house and home, or for a fun dessert with scoops of ice cream and strawberries.

The baked cookie dough has just the right texture to either break off bitesize pieces or cut into wedges.

175g/6 oz/¾ cup smooth peanut butter
175g/6 oz/¾ cup butter
1 tsp vanilla bean paste
225g/8 oz/1¾ cups plain (all-purpose) flour
150g/5½ oz/¾ cup soft light brown sugar
100g/3½ oz/½ cup caster (superfine) sugar
1 tsp bicarbonate of (baking) soda
1 egg, beaten
150g/5½ oz dark chocolate (70 per cent cocoa solids), chopped
75g/2¾ oz roasted unsalted peanuts, roughly chopped
½ tsp flaked sea salt, for sprinkling

Prep 35 minutes / **Cooking** 25 minutes / **Serves** 8–12

Heat the oven to 180°C/160°C fan/350°F/gas 4. Line a large baking tray with baking parchment and draw a circle about 25cm/10 inches in diameter as a guide.

Put the peanut butter, butter and vanilla in a saucepan and gently melt together, stirring with a spoon until smooth. Once melted, set aside to cool for about 10 minutes.

In a large bowl, combine the flour, sugars and bicarbonate of soda, then pour in the cooled peanut butter mixture. Add the egg, chocolate and peanuts, stirring gently until you have a ball of dough.

Press the dough onto the tray using the circle as a template. Sprinkle the salt over the top. Bake in the oven for 25 minutes until lightly golden.

Leave to cool on the lined tray for 5 minutes before serving warm as a soft-bake cookie or leave to cool completely until firm and crisp.

Flexible

Gluten-free: swap the flour for a plain gluten-free flour blend along with 1½ teaspoons xanthan gum.

Vegan: the butter can be substituted for a plant-based alternative. As for the egg, mix 1 tablespoon chia seeds with 3 tablespoons cold water. Leave for 10 minutes to thicken before using as you would the egg in the recipe.

*Flavour swap: for **cashew and white chocolate cookies**, simply swap the peanut butter and peanuts for the same weight of cashew butter and cashew nuts. Switch the dark chocolate with white chocolate.*

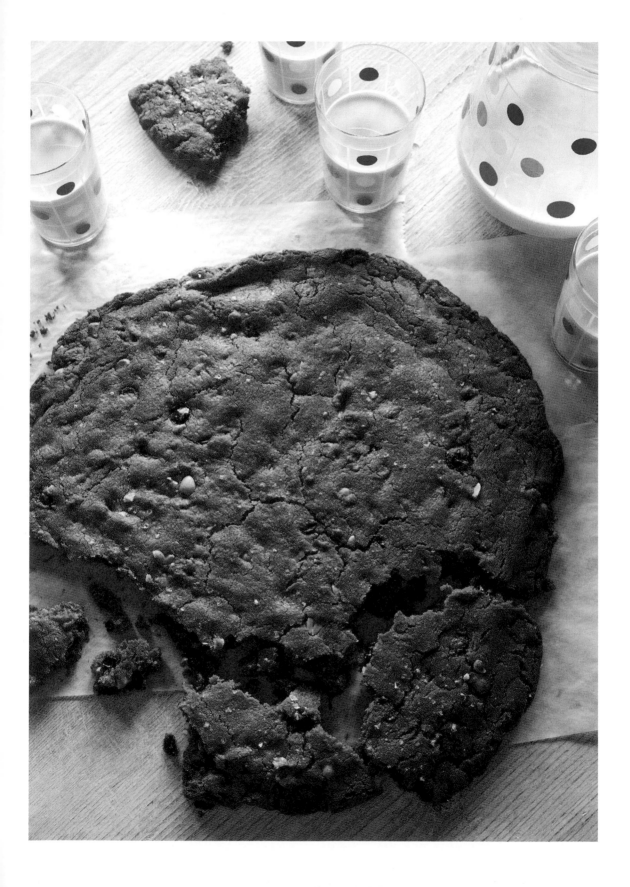

Coconut and sultana anzac biscuits

Anzac biscuits played a big part in my childhood, as whenever we went to visit my Nana, which was pretty much every week, she would always have a batch on the go. It was a recipe she could quickly throw together with basic everyday ingredients without any fussing about. Occasionally, she'd add in some sultanas or raisins, other times an additional spice. They were originally created as a robust biscuit with a long shelf life, that were sent to soldiers overseas in the early 1900's. This recipe makes plenty and even though I've tweaked these slightly to make them vegan friendly, they will still last weeks in an airtight container.

___

100g/3½ oz/¾ cup rolled oats

100g/3½ oz/¾ cup plain (all-purpose) flour

100g/3½ oz/½ cup caster (superfine) sugar

75g/2¾ oz/1 cup desiccated (shredded) coconut

75g/2¾ oz/½ cup sultanas (golden raisins)

½ tsp ground cinnamon

100g/3½ oz coconut oil

1 tbsp golden (corn) syrup

2 tbsp boiling water

1 tsp bicarbonate of (baking) soda

Prep 20 minutes / **Cooking** 10 minutes / **Makes** 20

Heat the oven to 180°C/160°C fan/350°F/gas 4. Line two baking trays with baking parchment.

Place the oats, flour, sugar, desiccated coconut, sultanas and cinnamon in a large mixing bowl and mix together.

Melt the coconut oil and golden syrup together in a saucepan.

Stir the water into the bicarbonate of soda and mix into to the coconut oil and syrup. Pour the mixture into the dry ingredients and mix until everything is combined. The mixture will be quite crumbly at this stage.

Spoon tablespoonfuls of the mixture onto the baking tray, spacing well apart to allow for spreading. I like to spoon and spread the mixture into an even layer in an 8cm/3¼ inch cookie cutter sitting on the tray, as it helps make even-sized biscuits. Bake for 10 minutes until golden. You may need to do this in batches. Once one batch has cooked, leave to cool on the trays for a couple of minutes before transferring to a wire rack to cool completely. Repeat with the remaining biscuit mixture.

Flexible

Gluten-free: *a standard gluten-free flour blend works well for these biscuits and make sure you use gluten-free oats.*

Flavour swap: *add 50g / 1¾ oz chopped dark chocolate or chopped hazelnuts when mixing all the dry ingredients together.*

*If you want to make the more classic **Anzac biscuits**, then swap the coconut oil for butter and omit the sultanas (golden raisins).*

Lemon and olive oil shortbread

My husband Phil has a weakness for shortbread, so he was my chief taste tester when putting this recipe together. I tried various versions that would be suitable for a variety of dietary requirements and still have the flexibility of using different flavours. These were the clear winner and are light, crisp and lemony. They should stay tasting fresh for a good few weeks once made, but if you have a Phil in your house then they won't be around long enough for you to check.

225g/8 oz/2¼ cups ground almonds

225g/8 oz/1½ cups polenta (cornmeal)

175g/6 oz/1¼ cups icing (confectioners') sugar, sifted

finely grated zest of 2 lemons

½ tsp flaked sea salt

225ml/8 fl oz/1 cup olive oil (avoid extra virgin olive oil as it's too flavoured)

1 tbsp caster (superfine) sugar

Prep 10 minutes / **Cooking** 50 minutes / **Makes** 16 pieces

Heat the oven to 170°C/150°C fan/325°F/gas 3.

Put the ground almonds, polenta, icing sugar, lemon zest and salt in a large bowl. Mix well to distribute the lemon zest. Add the olive oil and stir until everything is mixed together.

Transfer the dough to a round or square, 20cm/8 inch in diameter, cake tin and press into the edges, giving an even layer, about 2cm/¾ inches thick. Use a fork to create a pattern by pricking the dough and score out lines for cutting into portions when cooked.

Bake in the oven for 50 minutes, or until the surface is light golden and firm to touch.

As soon as it comes out of the oven, scatter with the caster sugar. Cut into portions or slices while warm, then leave to cool completely in the tin.

Flexible

Nut-free: *you can swap the ground almonds for the same amount of plain (all-purpose) flour or gluten-free flour. Bake as above.*

Flavour swap: *to make a **ginger shortbread**, omit the lemon zest from the mixture and instead add 75g/2¾ oz finely chopped stem ginger to the mix and continue to cook as above.*

*For a **coffee shortbread**, stir 4 tablespoons instant espresso powder into the dry mixture before adding the olive oil and omit the lemon.*

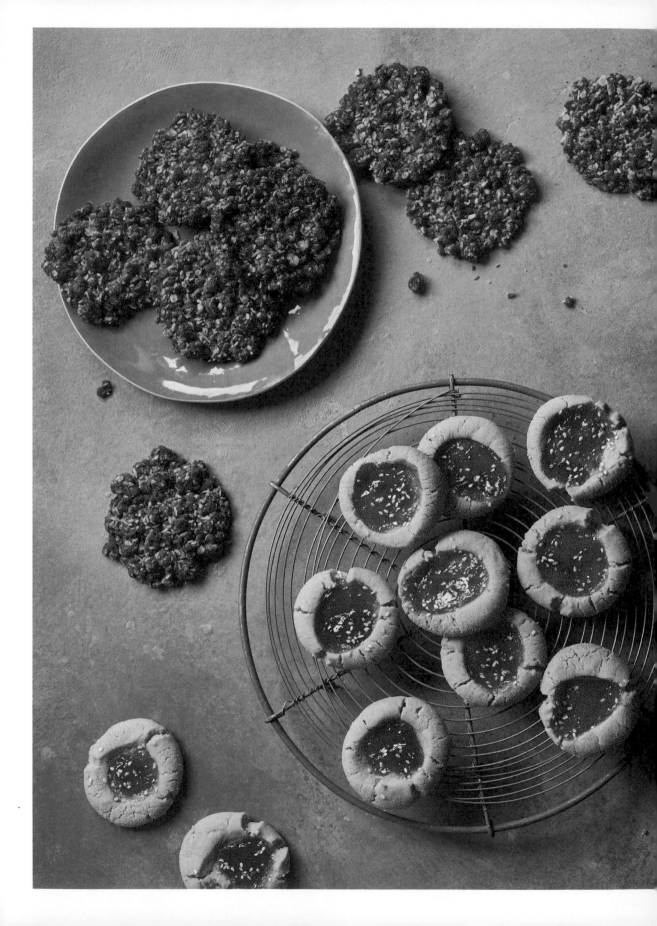

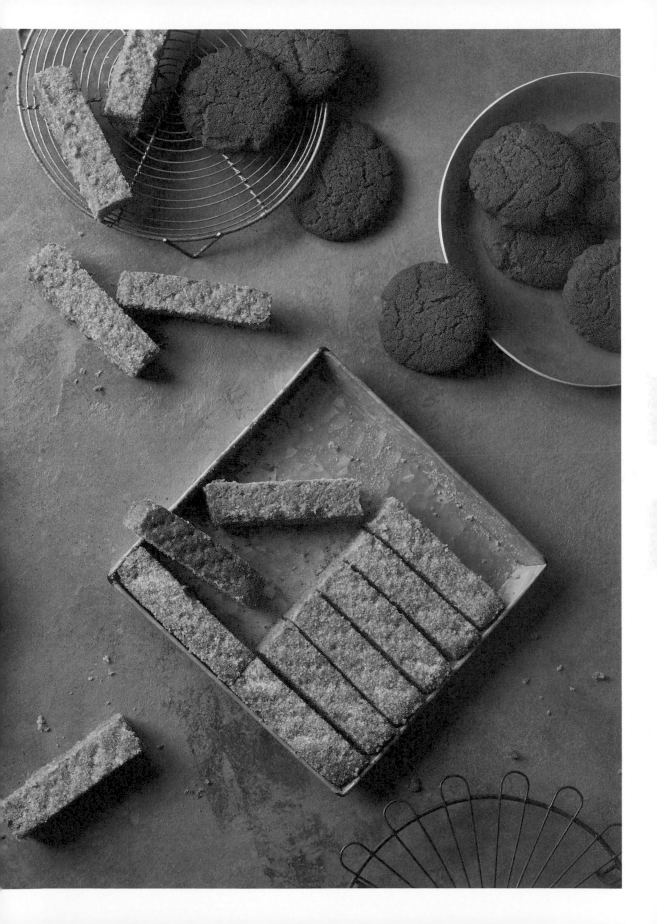

Ginger snap biscuits

You can't beat homemade ginger snap biscuits, and these are super gingery, as they use both dried ginger and plenty of fresh ginger for that extra hit. They have a beautiful crunchy texture and are dangerously addictive. I've my Grandma to thank for this recipe – I took it straight from her hand-written notebook of recipes she gave to me when I left home for university. She was such an enthusiastic cook and her ginger biscuits are one of many fantastic recipes I still make to this day. I'm sure she would be very proud to know this recipe is still going strong.

100g/1¾ oz/½ cup butter

85g/3 oz golden (corn) syrup

1½ tbsp grated fresh ginger

200g/7 oz/1½ cups self-raising
  (self-rising) flour

2 tbsp caster (superfine) sugar

2 tsp ground ginger

½ tsp ground cinnamon

1 tsp bicarbonate of (baking) soda

½ tsp flaked sea salt

Prep 25 minutes / **Cooking** 15 minutes / **Makes** 16

Heat the oven to 180°C/160°C fan/350°F/gas 4. Line two baking trays with baking parchment.

Put the butter, golden syrup and fresh ginger in a small saucepan and gently heat until the butter has melted. Set aside to cool for 5 minutes.

Mix together the flour, sugar, ground ginger, cinnamon, bicarbonate of soda and salt in a large bowl. Add the melted butter mixture and mix well to form a soft dough. Roll into 16 even-size balls and sit on the baking trays spaced apart to allow for some spreading. Flatten each one lightly with the palm of your hand.

Bake for 15 minutes until deep golden. Leave to cool on the trays for 5 minutes before transferring to a wire rack to cool completely.

Store in an airtight container for up to 2 weeks.

Flexible

Gluten-free: *use a gluten-free, self-raising (self-rising) flour blend along with ½ teaspoon xanthan gum. The end result is a little crumblier, so make sure they are totally cooled before removing from the tray.*

Flavour Swap: *For total ginger nuts, you can make **triple ginger snap biscuits**. Rather than 85g / 3oz golden (corn) syrup, use 40g / 1½ oz golden syrup and 40g / 1½ oz ginger syrup taken from a jar of stem ginger. Add to the butter along with the grated ginger and 1 finely chopped ball of stem ginger. Continue with the recipe as above.*

Tahini and apricot cookies

These are a Middle Eastern take on jammy thumbprint cookies using rich sesame seed paste and apricot jam. The addition of tahini not only gives them a crumbly, shortbread-like texture but makes them melt in the mouth. They take hardly any time at all to prepare and once made will stay fresh for days. If sesame isn't your thing, they can also be made using a smooth nut butter.

100g/3½ oz/½ cup butter, softened
75g/2¾ oz/⅓ cup caster (superfine) sugar
75g/2¾ oz tahini
½ tsp vanilla bean paste
150g/5½ oz/generous 1 cup plain (all-purpose) flour
1 tsp baking powder
3 tbsp apricot jam (jelly)
2 tsp sesame seeds

Prep 18 minutes / **Cooking** 12 minutes / **Makes** 16

Heat the oven to 180°C/160°C fan/350°F/gas 4. Line two baking trays with baking parchment.

Put the butter and sugar in a mixing bowl and beat together until light and creamy, either with an electric whisk or wooden spoon, depending on how energetic you're feeling.

Add the tahini and vanilla. Beat until smooth, then sift in the flour and baking powder. Mix until you have a smooth dough.

Roughly divide the dough into 16 pieces and roll into balls. Sit on the baking trays and press down in the middle of each one using your thumb, to make an imprint deep enough to fill with about ½ teaspoon apricot jam.

Fill each imprint with the jam and scatter over some sesame seeds. Bake in the oven for 12 minutes until the cookies are pale golden.

Leave to cool and firm up on the trays (removing them too early will cause them to crumble and break). Once cold, store in an airtight container.

Flexible

Gluten-free: simply swap the flour for a gluten-free flour and ½ teaspoon xanthan gum and make sure the baking powder is gluten-free.

*Flavour swap: to make **peanut butter and raspberry cookies**, swap the tahini for a smooth peanut butter (or any nut butter that takes your fancy), and use raspberry jam (jelly) in the middle instead of apricot.*

Sticky date and ginger cookies

There's something about these cookies that's deeply satisfying to eat. They're thick and chunky with a crisp outer and soft chewy middle. The dates create the stickiness in them and if you can, do try to use the Medjool dates – they taste like toffee.

300g/10½ oz/2¼ cups pitted dates, finely chopped
75g/3 oz stem ginger, finely chopped
175g/6 oz/¾ cup butter
150g/5½ oz/¾ cup soft light brown sugar
1 tbsp maple or golden (corn) syrup
½ tsp vanilla bean paste
300g/10½ oz/2¼ cups plain (all-purpose) flour
½ tsp baking powder
½ tsp grated nutmeg
½ tsp flaked sea salt

Prep 15 minutes / **Cooking** 12–14 minutes / **Makes** 14

Heat the oven to 180°C/160°C fan/350°F/gas 4. Line two baking trays with baking parchment.

Put the dates, ginger, butter, sugar, syrup and vanilla in a saucepan. Place the pan over a low heat, stirring until the butter has melted, sugar dissolved and dates starting to soften.

Sift together the flour, baking powder, nutmeg and salt into a large bowl. Add the date mixture and stir well until you have a wet dough.

Using an ice-cream scoop or a tablespoon, scoop balls of the dough and put on the lined baking trays, slightly spaced apart to allow room for spreading. Flatten the tops of each one by pressing lightly with the back of a fork.

Bake in the oven for 12–14 minutes until lightly golden. Leave to cool on the trays, and as they cool, they will firm up.

Once cooled completely, store in an airtight container.

Flexible

Vegan: *simply swap the butter for either coconut oil or a plant-based butter alternative.*

Gluten-free: *use a gluten-free flour and the addition of ½ teaspoon xanthan gum. Make sure the baking powder you use is also gluten-free.*

Flavour swap: *the finished cookies are delicious drizzled with melted dark or white chocolate.*

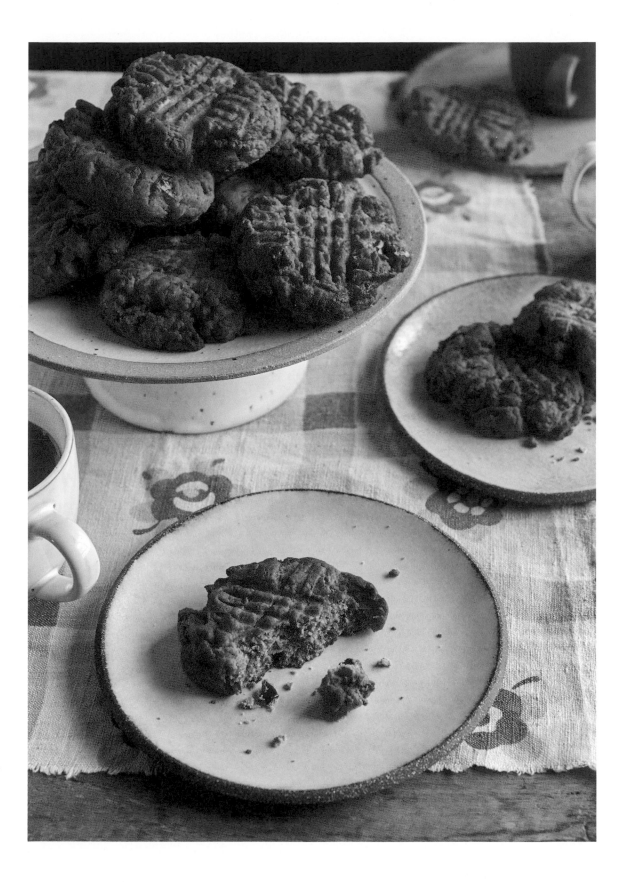

Chocolate brownie cookies

These indulgent cookies are a must for any chocolate fans with their shiny, cracked tops and rich, fudgy centres. The thick cookie dough is baked until it's just soft and chewy in the middle and then sprinkled with some flaked sea salt. Delicious eaten warm with a scoop of ice cream for dessert or just as they are at any time of the day.

225g/8 oz dark chocolate
  (70 per cent cocoa solids), chopped
75g/2¾ oz/⅓ cup butter
2 eggs
100g/3½ oz/½ cup caster (superfine)
  sugar
75g/2¾ oz/⅓ cup soft brown sugar
1 tsp vanilla bean paste
100g/3½ oz/¾ cup plain (all-purpose)
  flour
15g/½ oz cocoa powder
1 tsp baking powder
75g/2¾ oz/⅓ cup milk, dark or
  white chocolate chips
flaked sea salt, for sprinkling

Prep 25 minutes / **Cooking** 12–14 minutes / **Makes** 12

Heat the oven to 200°C/180°C fan/400°F/gas 6. Line two baking trays with baking parchment.

Put the dark chocolate and butter in a bowl over a pan of barely simmering water to slowly melt. Alternatively, gently melt in the microwave in 10-second bursts. One melted, set aside to cool for 10–15 minutes.

Whisk together the eggs, sugars and vanilla in a large bowl until light and frothy. Whisk in the cooled melted chocolate mixture until combined.

Sift the flour, cocoa powder and baking powder into the bowl, add the chocolate chips and stir everything together, giving you a thick cookie dough.

Using an ice-cream scoop or a tablespoon, scoop balls of the dough onto the lined baking trays, allowing a little room for spreading. Bake in the oven for 12–14 minutes, until they are starting to become firm on the outside but still a little soft in the middle.

As soon as they come out, scatter a little salt on the top of each one and leave to cool on the trays for a few minutes before eating warm or leaving to cool completely and storing in an airtight container.

Flexible

Gluten-free: *use a gluten-free flour blend and make sure the baking powder you use is also gluten-free. I have also made these with ground almonds instead of flour, which works well: the end result is slightly grainier and nuttier, but equally as delicious.*

Dairy-free: *swap the butter for a plant-based alternative, or for a coconutty flavour use coconut oil.*

Flavour swap: *you can really play around with flavours here such as adding grated orange zest, ground cinnamon or ground ginger to the mixture. Or you could substitute the chocolate chips for the same weight of chopped pecan nuts, dried cherries or cranberries.*

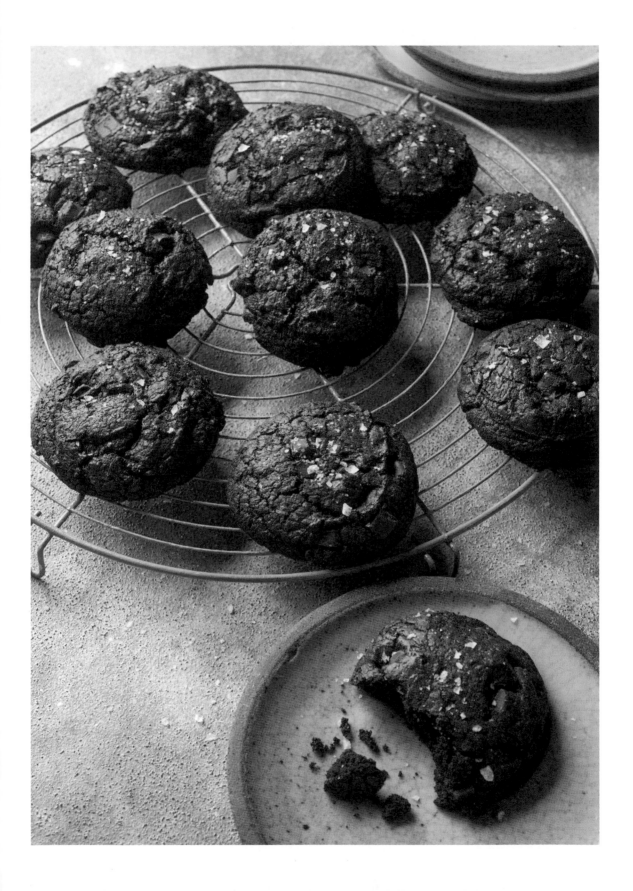

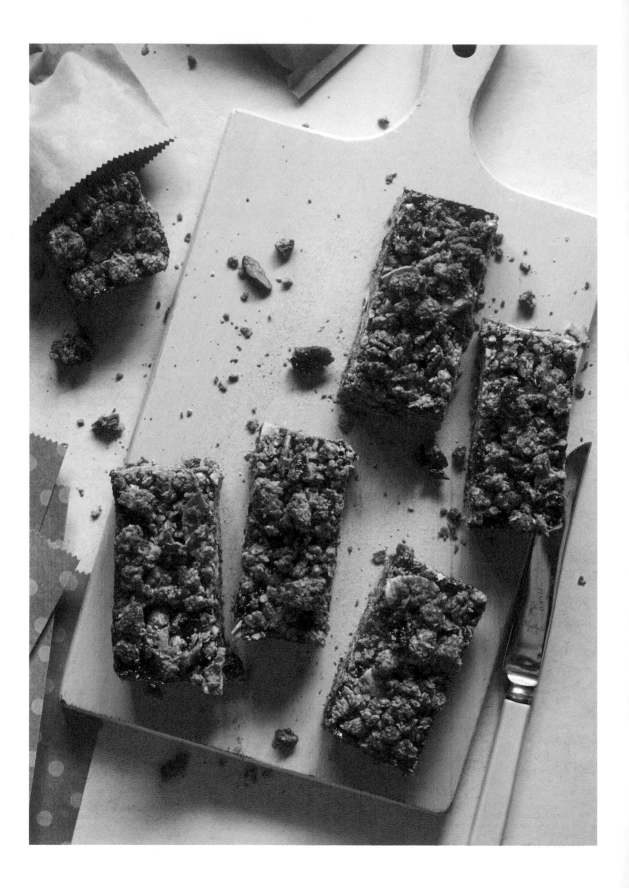

Berry granola bars

These are packed with all the good stuff we should be enjoying at breakfast for plenty of energy throughout the morning. The best thing about these bars is that you can customise them to create a flavour you love by switching around the dried berries, nuts, nut butter and jam. They're just perfect for an on-the-go breakfast or a portable snack.

225g/8 oz/1⅔ cups porridge (oatmeal) oats (gluten-free)

40g/1½ oz/scant ¼ cup soft light brown sugar

75g/2¾ oz dried cherries, cranberries or blueberries (or a mixture)

30g/1 oz flaked coconut

75g/2¾ oz/¾ cup pecan nuts, chopped

½ tsp flaked sea salt

½ tsp ground cinnamon

40g/1½ oz coconut oil

125g/4½ oz/½ cup cashew, almond, peanut or hazelnut nut butter

125ml/4 fl oz/½ cup maple syrup

75g/2¾ oz cherry or raspberry jam (jelly)

Prep 25 minutes / **Cooking** 20 minutes / **Makes** 10–12

Heat the oven to 180°C/160°C fan/350°F/gas 4. Line a 20 x 5 cm/ 8 x 2 inch baking tin with baking parchment.

Put 50g/1¾ oz/⅓ cup of the oats in a food processor and blitz until you have a fine powder that resembles flour. Transfer to a large mixing bowl and add the remaining oats, sugar, dried berries, coconut, pecans, salt and cinnamon. Briefly mix to combine.

Put the coconut oil, nut butter and maple syrup in a small saucepan and place over a gentle heat. Stir until everything has melted together. Pour this over the dry ingredients and mix well, so everything is coated in the syrupy nut butter.

Transfer the granola mixture into the prepared tin, keeping a large handful back in the bowl. Press firmly into the base and sides using the back of a spoon. Spoon over the jam and spread over the surface. Finish by scattering the reserved granola on top.

Bake for 20 minutes or until golden and crunchy on top. Allow to cool in the tin before turning out onto a board and cutting into bars. Keeps for up to 1 week in an airtight container.

Flexible

*Flavour swap: to make **apricot and chocolate chip granola bars**, use 75g/2¾ oz/½ cup chopped apricots in place of the berries and stir in 75g/2¾ oz dark chocolate chips (dairy-free if you are vegan) into the granola, and top with apricot jam (jelly) instead of a berry jam (jelly).*

*To make **honey, sultana and almond granola bars**, use 75g/2¾ oz/½ cup sultanas (golden raisins) in place of the berries and 75g/2¾ oz/⅔ cup chopped almonds in place of the pecan nuts. Rather than maple syrup, use the same amount of honey. Do note, this isn't suitable for vegans if using honey.*

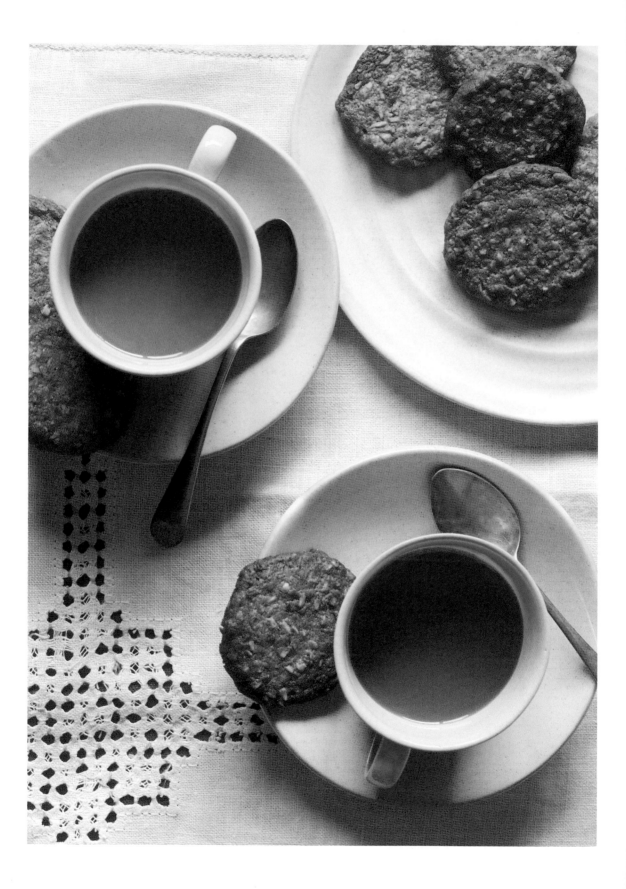

Buckwheat, hazelnut and orange butter biscuits

These biscuits are delicate, crisp and buttery, and would be great to serve with creamy desserts such as a posset or syllabub. I find myself sneaking the odd one here and there throughout the day if I've made a batch, but they are light and delicate enough to not feel guilty about!

They use buckwheat flour, which is naturally gluten-free and has a very distinctive strong nutty flavour.

100g/3½ oz/½ cup butter, chilled
  and diced
75g/2¾ oz/scant ½ cup toasted hazelnuts,
  finely chopped
75g/2¾ oz/½ cup buckwheat flour
¼ tsp flaked sea salt
50g/1¾ oz/¼ cup caster (superfine) sugar
finely grated zest of 1 orange
1 egg yolk

Prep 20 minutes, plus 1 hour chilling / **Cooking** 15 minutes / **Makes** 20

Put the butter, hazelnuts, flour and salt in a mixing bowl and rub with your fingers until you have a coarse crumb texture. Add the sugar and orange zest and mix well before stirring in the egg yolk and mixing until you have a dough.

Shape the dough into a log shape around 5 x 25cm/2 x 10 inches long and wrap in a piece of cling film. Put in the fridge to chill for about 1 hour.

Heat the oven to 180°C/160°C fan/350°F/gas 4. Line two baking trays with baking parchment.

Remove the cling film from the dough and using a sharp knife, cut into 5mm/¼ inch slices. Lay on the baking trays, spaced well apart to allow for spreading.

Bake for 15 minutes or until light golden. Leave to cool on the trays, then store in an airtight container for up to 1 week.

Flexible

Vegan: *you won't get such a rich flavour as dairy butter, but you can use a plant-based butter alternative in these biscuits. To replace the egg yolk, mix 2 teaspoons ground flaxseed with 1 tablespoon cold water. Leave for 5 minutes to thicken before mixing into the dry biscuit ingredients.*

Flavour swap: *chopped almonds, macadamia nuts or desiccated (shredded) coconut can all be used as an alternative to the hazelnuts. Rather than orange zest, you can swap for grapefruit, lemon or lime zest.*

Flour swap: *if gluten-free flour isn't a requirement to you, then standard wheat flours can be used. I particularly like spelt flavour as it has a mild nutty flavour that ties well with the rest of the ingredients.*

Pistachio, apricot and dark chocolate biscotti

These twice-baked crisp Italian biscuits are a fantastic after-dinner coffee accompaniment, or low-fat pick-me-up throughout the day. The colourful pistachios, apricots and dark chocolate are a great combination, however, other dried fruits, nuts and chocolate chips work just as well in the biscotti, so don't feel you have to stick to the recipe.

225g/8 oz/1¾ cups plain (all-purpose) flour, plus more for dusting

1½ tsp baking powder

175g/6 oz/scant 1 cup caster (superfine) sugar

finely grated zest of 1 orange

nutmeg, for grating

2 eggs, beaten

75g/2¾ oz pistachio nuts

75g/2¾ oz dried apricots, finely chopped

75g/2¾ oz dark chocolate chips

Prep 15 minutes / **Cooking** 55 minutes / **Makes** 24

Heat the oven to 180°C/160°C fan/350°F/gas mark 4. Line a large baking tray with baking parchment.

Put the flour, baking powder, sugar, orange zest and a good grating of nutmeg in a large bowl and mix to combine. Add the eggs and when the mixture starts to come together, use your hands to form a sticky dough. Add the pistachios, apricots and chocolate, working the dough so they are evenly distributed.

Dust your work surface with flour, and you may find it helpful to dust your hands lightly with flour too, as the dough will be a little sticky. Divide the dough in half and roughly shape each one into oval log shapes, about 5 x 25cm/2 x 10 inch.

Place the logs on the baking tray, spaced apart, and cook for 25–30 minutes, or until the dough has risen, spread and is almost firm but still pale in colour.

Transfer the loaves to a wire rack and leave for 5 minutes to cool and firm up some more. Reduce the oven to 150°C/130°C fan/300°F/gas 2. Using a serrated knife, cut each baked loaf diagonally into fingers about 1cm/¼ inch thick.

Lay the biscotti flat onto the baking trays in a single layer and cook for another 15 minutes, turn over and cook for a further 10 minutes until golden and crisp. Cool on a wire rack and then store them in an airtight container. They should stay crisp for up to 4 weeks.

Flexible

Vegan: Combine 100ml / 3½ fl oz aquafaba (liquid from tinned chickpeas) and 2 tablespoons smooth nut butter. Mix and use in place of the eggs in the recipe. Make sure you use dairy-free chocolate chips.

Gluten-free: use a gluten-free flour and add 1 teaspoon xanthan gum. Take care when slicing the biscotti after the first bake as it will be more crumbly than when using wheat flour.

Nut-free: swap the nuts for additional dried fruit, such as figs, cherries or cranberries.

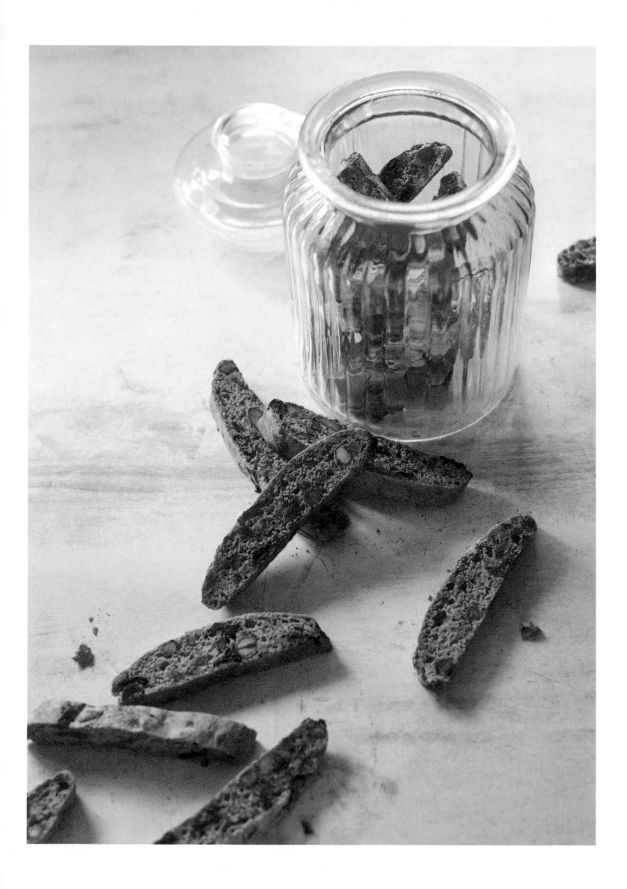

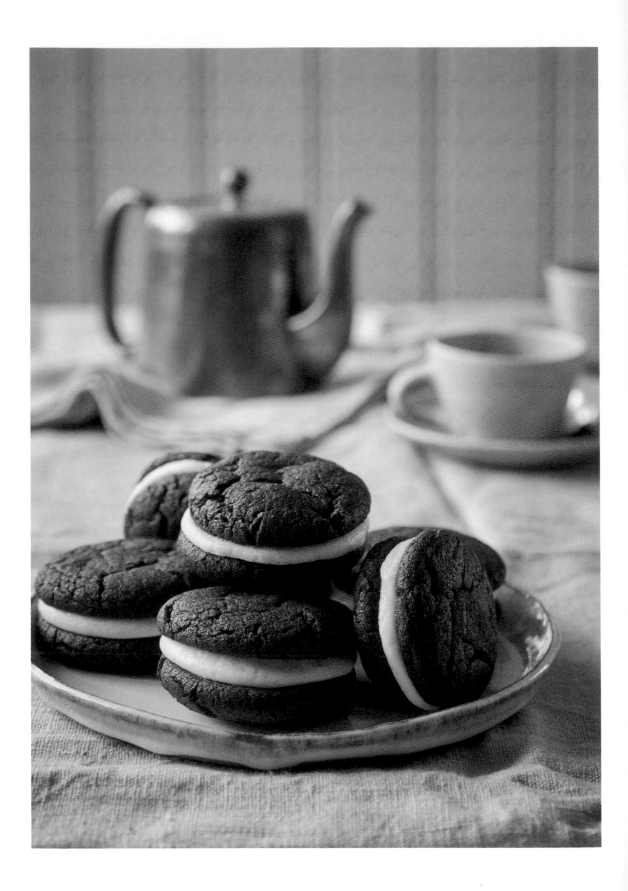

Chocolate and peppermint cookie creams

If, like me, you love the flavour combination of chocolate and mint then you'll love these. Not only do the chocolate cookies themselves have a lovely light crisp texture, but when sandwiched together with the peppermint filling it is like biting into a sweet fluffy minty cloud.

I prefer to pipe the mint filling as it makes the process far quicker and the end result neater, though you can just spread it on with a knife if you prefer.

For the cookies
150g/5½ oz/⅔ cup butter, softened
100g/3½ oz/½ cup soft brown sugar
150g /5½ oz golden (corn) syrup
200g/7 oz/1½ cups plain (all-purpose) flour
50g/1¾ oz/½ cup cocoa powder
1 tsp bicarbonate of (baking) soda

For the filling
250g/9 oz/1¾ cups icing (confectioners') sugar, sifted
3 tbsp milk
35g/1¼ oz butter, softened
½–1 tsp peppermint extract
2 tbsp crushed hard mint sweets (candies) such as candy canes (optional)

Prep 15 minutes, plus 30 minutes chilling / **Cooking** 12 minutes / **Makes** 12–14

To make the cookies, in a large bowl beat together the butter, sugar and golden syrup with an electric whisk for a few minutes until light and fluffy. Sift in the flour, cocoa powder and bicarbonate of soda and mix together to form a thick cookie dough. Put into the fridge for about 30 minutes to firm up.

Meanwhile make the filling. Beat together the icing sugar, milk and butter until light and creamy, then add ½ teaspoon peppermint extract. If you want a strong minty flavour, add in the other ½ teaspoon. Stir through the crushed mints, if using, for a crunch.

Heat the oven to 180°C/160°C fan/350°F/gas 4. Line two baking trays with baking parchment.

Once the cookie dough has firmed up, scoop tablespoons of it into balls, giving you 24–28 in total, making sure you have an even number. Sit on the baking trays, spaced apart to allow for spreading, and bake for 10–12 minutes until they are cracked on top.

Remove from the oven and leave on the trays to firm up before transferring to a wire rack to cool completely.

Spread a heaped dessertspoon of the filling on the underside of half of the cookies, then sandwich together with the remaining cookies, pressing lightly to stick together. Store in an airtight container.

Flexible

Vegan: switch the butter for a plant-based alternative in the cookie mix, and use a plant-based milk for the peppermint filling.

Flavour swap: you can really play around with the flavour of the cookie filling here:

Orange: use orange extract or grated zest of 1 orange in place of peppermint extract.

Peanut butter: swap the butter for a crunchy or smooth peanut butter and omit the peppermint extract.

Tahini: swap the butter for tahini and omit the peppermint extract. Sprinkle the biscuits with some sesame seeds before baking.

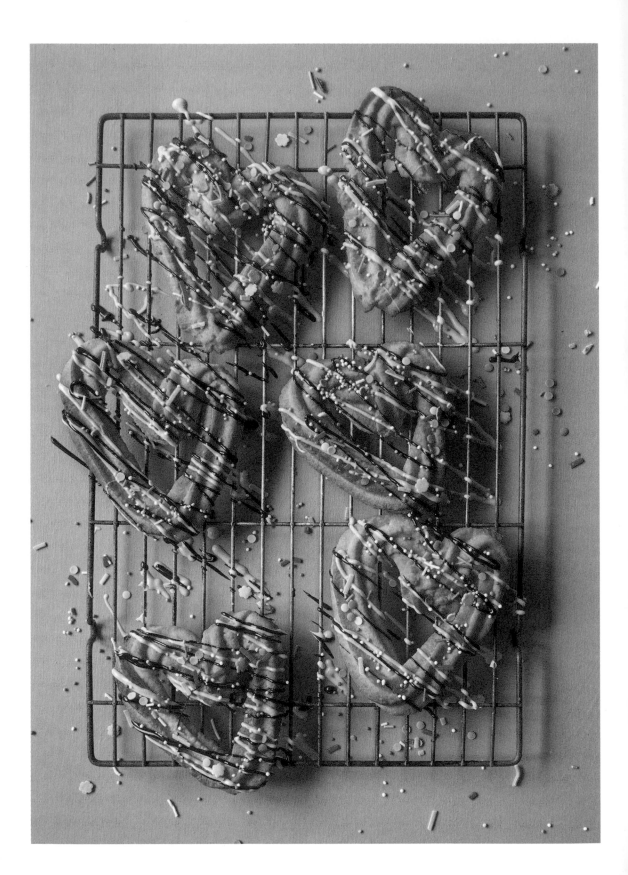

Viennese hearts

These versatile biscuits can be made as per the main recipe or easily swapped to be vegan, gluten-free, chocolate or lemon flavoured or piped into different shapes. They are fun to make especially if you have an occasion to bake for whether it's a birthday, valentines or simply to say 'I love you'. I like to finish them off drizzled with chocolate, but a lemon or orange glacé icing would be just as good, should you prefer.

For the cookies

125g/4½ oz/½ cup butter, softened

125g/4½ oz/1 cup plain (all-purpose) flour

40g/1½ oz icing/¼ cup (confectioners') sugar

25g/1 oz ground almonds

25g/1 oz cornflour (cornstarch)

1 tsp vanilla bean paste

1–2 tsp milk (optional)

To decorate

25g/1 oz dark, milk or white chocolate coloured sprinkles (optional)

Prep 30 minutes / **Cooking** 12–15 minutes / **Makes** 8–10

Heat the oven to 180°C/160°C fan/350°F/gas 4. Line two baking trays with baking parchment.

Put the butter in a food processor or mixer and beat until it's very soft. Add the flour, icing sugar, ground almonds, cornflour and vanilla. Beat together until smooth and soft. It needs to be a pipeable consistency but still able to hold its shape. If you think it's too firm, beat in 1–2 teaspoons milk.

Transfer the biscuit dough to a large piping bag with a large star nozzle. Pipe heart shapes (or any shape you like such as fingers, circles, letters or numbers) and bake for 12–15 minutes until lightly golden brown.

Cool on the tray for a few minutes before carefully lifting onto a wire rack to cool completely.

To decorate the biscuits, place the chocolate in a bowl over a pan of barely simmering water to slowly melt. Alternatively, gently melt in the microwave in 10-second bursts. Transfer the melted chocolate to a small piping bag with a thin nozzle, then drizzle chocolate over the top of the biscuits. Scatter with any sprinkles while the chocolate is still warm, if using. Leave to set before serving.

Flexible

***Gluten-free:** replace the flour with a gluten-free flour and add 1 teaspoon xanthan gum. These are a little more delicate than with wheat flour but have a wonderful melt-in-the-mouth texture.*

***Vegan:** use a plant-based margarine in place of the butter, and make sure you use a dairy-free-chocolate to decorate.*

***Flavour swap:** to make **chocolate hearts**, replace 30g/1 oz of the plain (all-purpose) flour with sifted cocoa powder. Drizzle with melted chocolate and decorate with chocolate sprinkles.*

*To make **lemon hearts**, swap the vanilla bean paste for the finely grated zest of 1 lemon. Decorate with a lemon glacé icing made from 40g/1½ oz cup/¼ cup icing (confectioners') sugar mixed with 1½ tsp lemon juice to make a thin runny icing.*

Coffee and almond macaroons

The word macaroons can cause plenty of confusion. These are the English-style ones and very different to the delicate colourful French ones. They're crisp and cracked on the outside with a slightly soft chewiness in the middle and are ridiculously quick and simple to make. Enjoy with coffee, or as an accompaniment to light desserts such as chocolate mousse. As they last for ages once baked, they make fantastic gifts when wrapped in cellophane bags tied with a ribbon or packed into small boxes.

125g/4½ oz/1¼ cups ground almonds
150g/5½ oz/¾ cup caster (superfine) sugar
2 tbsp instant espresso powder
2 egg whites
18–20 blanched almonds

Prep 15 minutes / **Cooking** 16–18 minutes / **Makes** 18–20

Heat the oven to 180°C/160°C fan/350°F/gas 4. Line a baking tray with baking parchment.

Mix together the ground almonds, sugar and espresso powder in a large bowl. In a separate bowl, whisk the egg whites until they are becoming foamy, but not yet holding their shape.

Fold the egg whites into the almond mixture until you have a sticky dough.

Using wet hands so the dough doesn't stick, roll the mixture into 18–20 small balls and place on the baking tray, spaced 2 finger widths apart to allow for spreading. Lightly press an almond onto the centre of each one.

Bake for 16–18 minutes until they are firm but feel like they are a little soft in the middle, taking care not to overbake them. They want to be slightly chewy inside still.

Cool on the trays for a few minutes before transferring to a wire rack to completely cool. Store in an airtight container for up to 2 weeks.

Flexible

*Flavour swap: to make **cardamom and pistachio macaroons**, replace 60g / 2 oz / ⅔ cup of the ground almonds with pistachio nuts. Blitz them to a fine powder in a mini blender and swap the espresso powder for ½ teaspoon ground cardamom. Top each one with a pistachio before baking.*

*To make **festive macaroons**, replace the espresso powder with ½ teaspoon mixed (apple pie) spice and finely grated zest of 1 small orange. When cool, dip the bases in 75g / 2¾ oz melted dark chocolate and leave to set.*

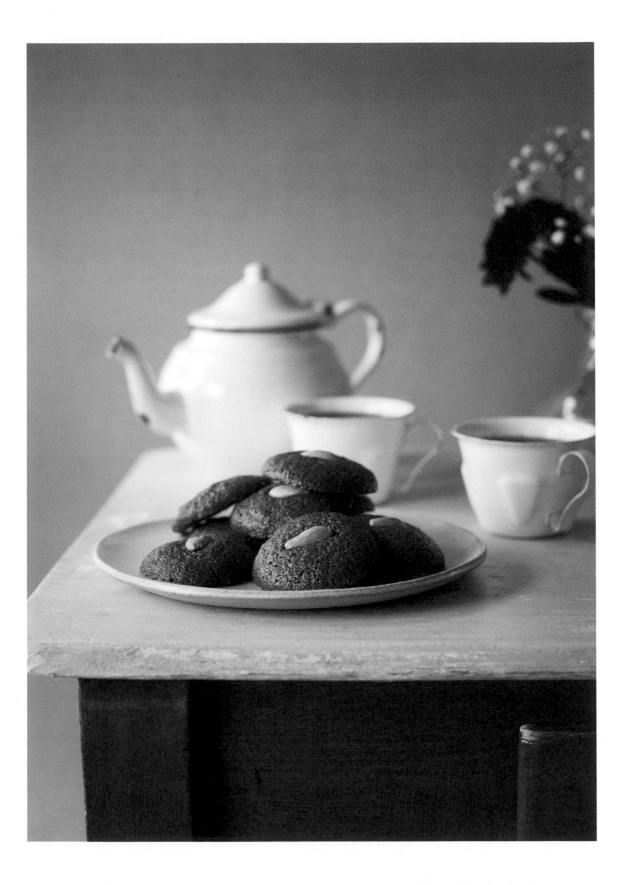

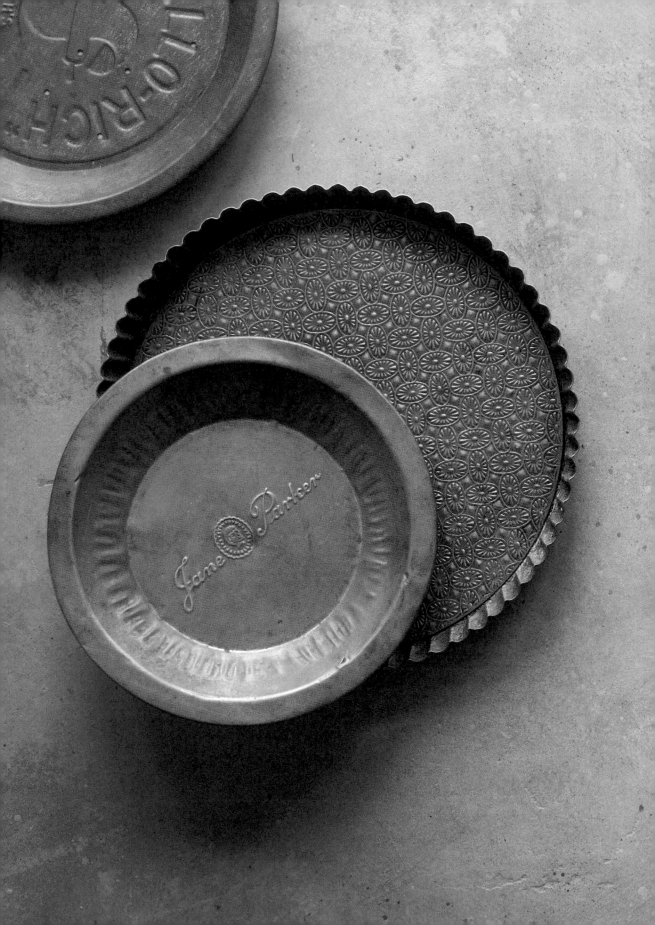

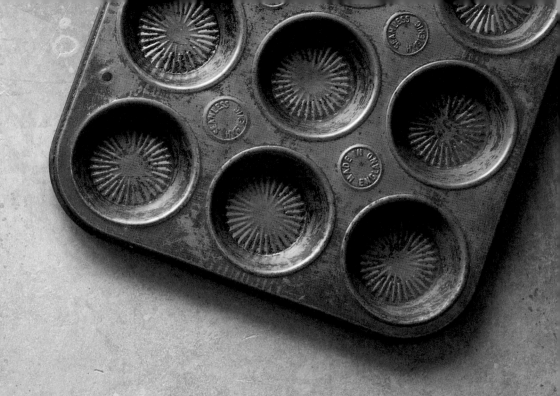

pastries

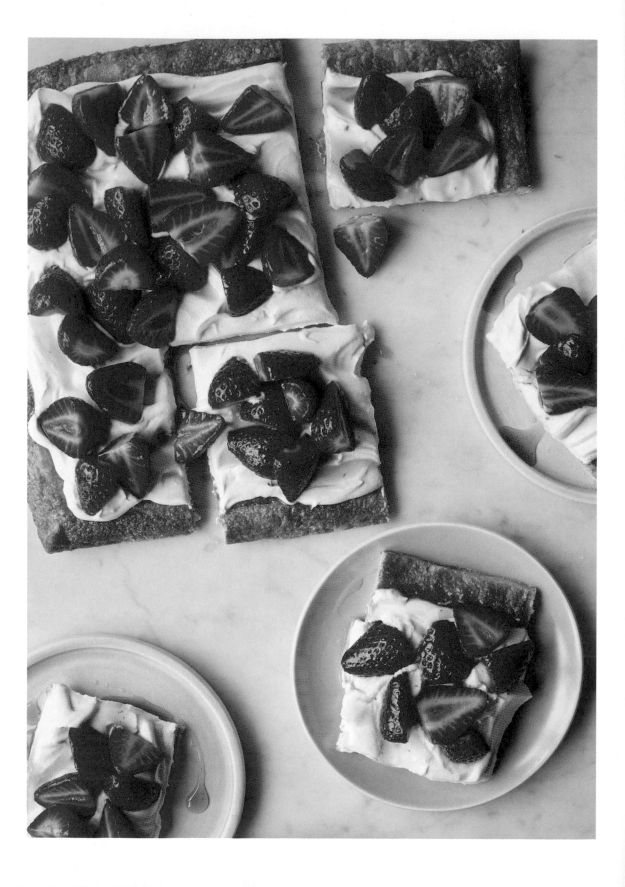

Strawberry cheesecake tart

Sometimes simplicity is best and when fresh strawberries are at their sweetest and juiciest, there is very little they need to be served with. The crunchy puff pastry base and sweet mascarpone cream are all that is required here. The fact that this is so simple to make is an absolute bonus – and you can easily fool any dinner guests into thinking you've spent hours making it just for them!

When strawberries are not so great, I would go for other fruits such as slices of ripe peaches or nectarines and some raspberries, or why not try one of my Flexible suggestions below.

320g/11 oz sheet ready rolled puff pastry
1 egg, beaten, for glazing
75g/2¾ oz/⅓ cup caster (superfine) sugar,
   plus 2 tbsp for sprinkling
450g/1 lb strawberries
200g/7 oz/scant 1 cup mascarpone cheese
100g/3½ oz/scant ½ cup natural yoghurt
1 tsp vanilla bean paste
125ml/4 fl oz/½ cup double (heavy) cream
icing (confectioners') sugar,
   for dusting (optional)

Prep 20 minutes / **Cooking** 20 minutes / **Serves** 6–8

Heat the oven to 200°C/180°C fan/400°F/gas 6. Line a large baking tray with baking parchment.

Place the pastry on the tray and using a small sharp knife, score a 2cm/¾ inch border around the edge. Prick the inside several times with a fork. Brush the pastry all over with egg and sprinkle with the 2 tablespoons sugar.

Bake for 20 minutes or until the pastry is puffed and golden. Set aside to cool. As it cools the pastry will flatten.

While the pastry is cooking, cut the strawberries in half, or quarters if they are big, and toss in 50g/1¾ oz/¼ cup of the sugar. Leave to macerate for around 15 minutes or so to become juicy.

To make the cheesecake cream, beat together the mascarpone, yoghurt, remaining 25g/1 oz sugar and vanilla until smooth.

In a separate bowl, whisk the cream until it forms soft peaks, then fold through the mascarpone mixture. Spoon over the top of the pastry, then spoon over the strawberries and any juices. Finish with a dusting of icing sugar, if liked, to serve.

Flexible

Flavour swap: *the strawberries can be swapped for any other fresh berries. Or why not try:*

Mango, lime and passion fruit tart: *swap the vanilla for the grated zest of 1 lime. Swap the strawberries for 2 ripe mangoes, cut into chunks and mixed with the pulp from 2 ripe passion fruit.*

Rhubarb and custard tart: *swap the yoghurt for 100ml/ 3½ fl oz ready-made custard. Top the tart with 400g/14 oz cooked rhubarb (see page 102 for a nice way to roast rhubarb) and finish with a dusting of icing sugar.*

Key lime cream puffs

This may appear to be a complicated recipe but believe me, it's not. First up, the lime curd can be made in advance and kept in the fridge. It's tangier and tastier than shop bought, but if you are pushed for time, then grab a good-quality jar instead as an alternative.

The buns are made with choux pastry. The key with this is to make sure they are thoroughly cooked through, otherwise they will go soggy when removed from the oven. Finally, the mascarpone cream, which is a doddle to make. They are delicate and irresistible.

For the curd
finely grated zest and juice of 2 limes
100g/3½ oz/½ cup caster (superfine) sugar
2 eggs
50g/1¾ oz butter, diced and
  room temperature

For the pastry
50g/1¾ oz butter
70g/2½ oz/½ cup plain (all-purpose)
  flour, sifted
2 eggs, beaten

For the cream
125g/4½ oz/½ cup mascarpone cheese
40g/1½ oz/¼ cup icing (confectioners')
  sugar, sifted
1 tsp vanilla bean paste
125ml/4 fl oz/½ cup double (heavy) cream

To decorate
75g/2¾ oz white chocolate, chopped
icing (confectioners') sugar, for dusting

Prep 1 hour / **Cooking** 30 minutes / **Makes** 16–18

To make the lime curd, whisk together the lime juice, zest, sugar and eggs in a heavy-based saucepan. Place over a low-medium heat and stir continuously until slightly thickened. Whisk in a little butter at a time, cook and stir for around 5 minutes until you have a smooth, thick lime curd. Transfer to a bowl and leave to cool.

Heat the oven to 200°C/180°C fan/400°F/gas 6. Line two baking trays with baking parchment and spray or splash with a little water.

For the pastry, put the butter and 150ml/5½ fl oz/⅔ cup water in a medium saucepan over a low heat. Once the butter has melted, bring slowly to the boil, tip in the flour and beat vigorously. Once the mixture becomes a smooth paste that forms a ball, continue stirring for a few minutes before removing from the heat. Leave to cool for 3–4 minutes, then add the eggs to the paste a little at a time, beating well, until the mixture is thick, smooth and glossy.

Spoon into a large piping bag fitted with a 1cm/½ inch plain nozzle. Pipe 3–4cm/1¼–1½ inch dollops of the mixture onto the baking trays, leaving a little room between each one for them to spread. Flatten any peaks with a wet finger for a smooth finish.

Bake for 30 minutes until well risen and golden brown. Once they are out of the oven and cool enough to handle, using a serrated knife, cut the top third off each one to allow the steam to escape and transfer them to a wire rack to cool completely.

For the cream, beat the mascarpone, sugar and vanilla until smooth. Whisk in the cream until it is thick and pipeable, then transfer to a piping bag with a plain or star nozzle. Pipe some mascarpone cream into each puff and top with a teaspoon of lime curd. Sit the cut piece of pastry on top. Melt the chocolate in a bowl over a pan of barely simmering water then drizzle over the top of the puffs and finish with a dusting of icing sugar. Serve immediately.

Flexible

Gluten-free: for the choux pastry you can use a gluten-free flour blend with the addition of ¼ teaspoon xanthan gum and cook in the same way as above.

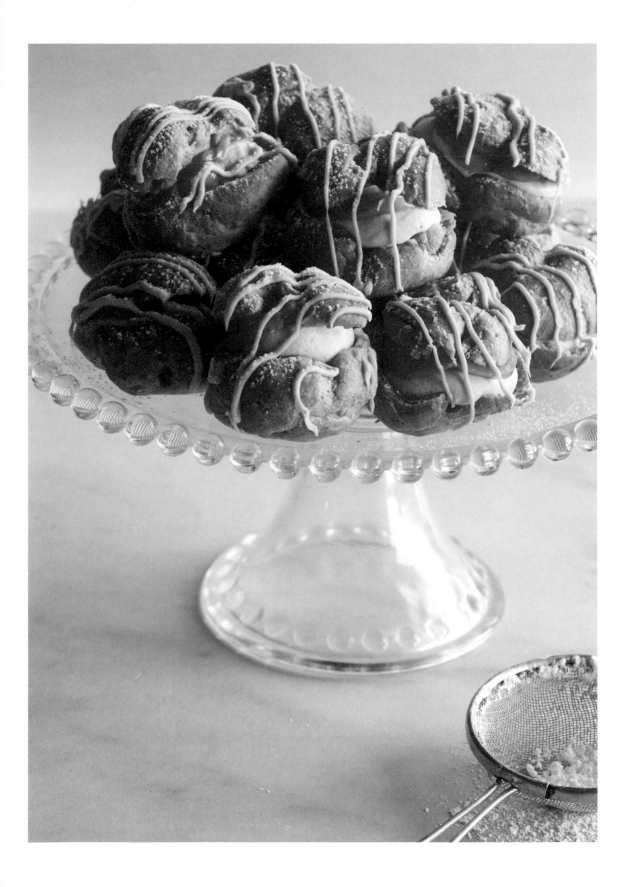

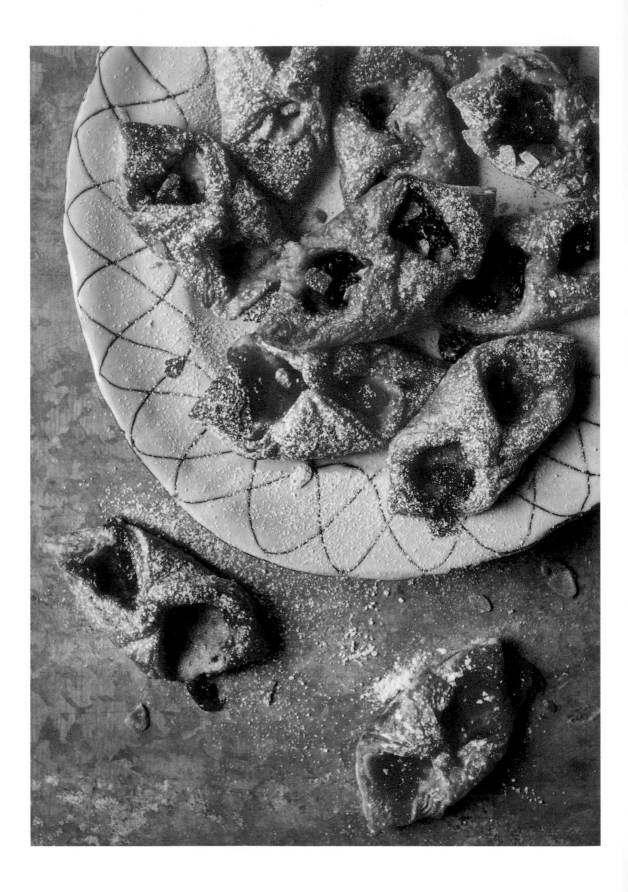

Prepare-ahead breakfast pastries

These are the perfect make-ahead breakfast that can be stored in the freezer so you can enjoy freshly baked pastries whenever you like. Made with individual portions of puff pastry, layer of sweetened cream cheese and a dollop of your chosen jam, they are a quick to make, quick to cook and especially quick to eat!

320g/11 oz sheet ready rolled puff pastry

100g/3½ oz/scant ½ cup mascarpone cheese

40g/1½ oz/scant ¼ cup caster (superfine) sugar

1 tbsp maple syrup or honey

1 tsp vanilla bean paste

3 tbsp of your favourite fruit jam (jelly)

1 egg yolk, mixed with 1 tbsp milk (egg wash)

2 tbsp flaked (slivered) almonds (optional)

3 tbsp icing (confectioners') sugar, plus extra for dusting

Prep 30 minutes / **Cooking** 15–18 minutes / **Makes** 12

Line a baking tray that will fit in your freezer with baking parchment. Unroll the pastry and cut into 12 squares, then transfer the pastry to the baking tray and make a start on the filling.

Beat together the mascarpone, sugar, maple syrup or honey and vanilla until completely smooth. Transfer to a piping bag and pipe about 1 tablespoon in the middle of each pastry square. Alternatively, you can use a spoon and dollop in the middle of the pastry.

Spoon a teaspoon of your chosen jam on top of the filling and brush the pastry with the egg wash. Scatter over the flaked almonds, if using, and dust with icing sugar. Now pull up 2 opposite corners of the pastry and gently pinch and twist to seal on top of the filling. Put the baking tray in the freezer. After a couple of hours, or when the pastries are totally frozen, you can transfer them to a freezer bag to store.

When you are ready to cook the pastries, heat the oven to 200°C/180°C fan/400°F/gas 6. Sit the pastries in a single layer on a baking tray lined with baking parchment and bake on a low shelf in the oven for 15–18 minutes until puffed and golden.

Cool for 10 minutes then dust with icing sugar, if preferred, before serving warm or they can be left to cool completely and served cold – either way, they are best eaten the day they are baked.

Flexible

Vegan: make sure you use a vegan puff pastry. Swap the mascarpone for a plant-based cream cheese alternative. Brush the tops with some plant-based milk rather than the egg wash.

Gluten-free: a gluten-free puff pastry will work well in this recipe.

Cherry turnovers

Golden, flaky and simply irresistible, enjoy these fruity turnovers while still warm with a dusting of icing sugar, or leave to cool and you have portable mini cherry pies to enjoy any time of the day.

You can freeze the assembled turnovers before baking and when ready to cook, brush with the cream and sprinkle with sugar, adding a further 5 minutes to your cooking time.

For the pastry

275g/9¾ oz/2 cups plain (all-purpose) flour, plus extra for dusting

175g/6 oz/¾ cup butter, chilled and diced

2 tsp caster (superfine) sugar, plus 1 tbsp for sprinkling

1 tsp fine sea salt

125–150ml/4–5 fl oz/½–⅔ cup ice-cold water

30ml/2 tbsp double (heavy) cream

For the filling

300g/10½ oz pitted cherries, fresh or frozen (defrosted if frozen), roughly chopped

40g/1½ oz butter

3 tbsp caster (superfine) sugar

½ tsp almond essence (optional)

1½ tsp cornflour (cornstarch), mixed with 1 tbsp water to make a paste

Prep 25 minutes, plus 30 minutes resting / **Cooking** 25 minutes / **Makes** 9

To make the pastry, put the flour, butter, sugar and salt in a large bowl. Using your fingers, roughly rub in the butter, leaving large chunks than for shortcrust, to give a flakier pastry. Drizzle over 125ml/4 fl oz/½ cup of the water and bring together with your hands, using the remaining water if required. Shape into a ball, wrap in cling film and put in the fridge for 30 minutes.

While the pastry is chilling, put the cherries, butter, sugar and almond essence, if using, in a saucepan over a medium heat. Cook for 10 minutes, stirring occasionally, until the cherries are soft. Add the cornflour paste and stir until slightly thickened. Transfer to a bowl and chill. The cherry filling should be cool before using.

Heat the oven to 200°C/180°C fan/400°F/gas 6. Line 2 baking trays with baking parchment and dust with flour.

Dust the worktop with flour. Remove the pastry from the fridge and roll out until it's around 3mm/⅛ inch thick. Cut into 9 even squares, about 14cm x 14cm/5½ inches, re-rolling any trimmings to use up the pastry.

Spoon a heaped tablespoon of the filling in the middle of each pastry piece. Brush the edges with water and fold the pastry over. Seal by crimping firmly with a fork and pierce a hole in the top of each one with the tip of a sharp knife.

Transfer the turnovers to the baking trays, and brush over the top of each one with the cream. Sprinkle with the remaining sugar and bake for 25 minutes, until golden brown. Cool for about 10 minutes before serving (very important as the filling is extremely hot!) or cool on a wire rack and serve at room temperature.

Flexible

Vegan: *use a plant-based butter for the pastry and to make the filling, and a plant-based cream for brushing the turnovers before baking.*

Flavour swap: *for **peach turnovers** swap the cherries for peeled and diced fresh or tinned peaches. Cook the filling as above, until it's a thick compote consistency then cool. Use 2 teaspoons of filling for each pastry and top with a couple of peach slices. Fold, seal and bake as above.*

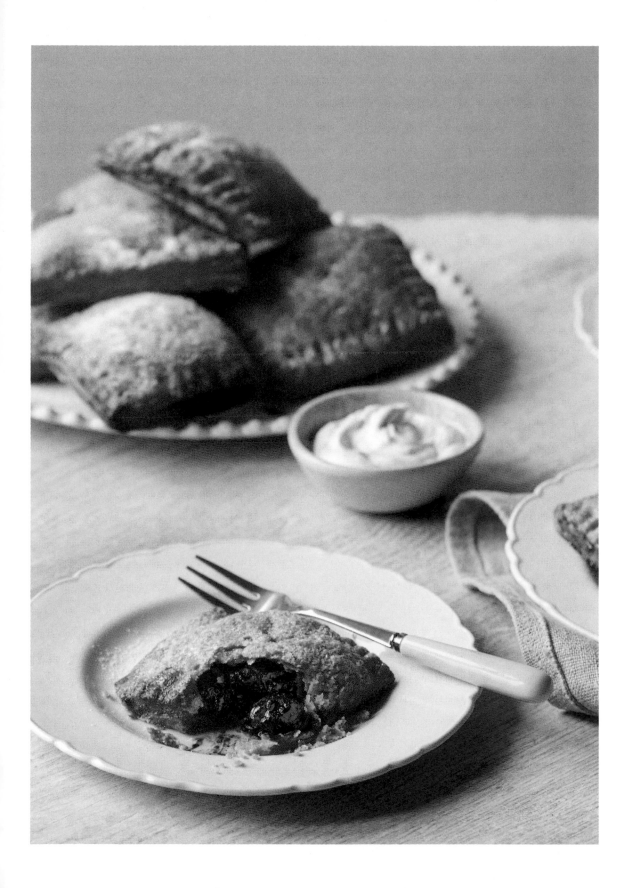

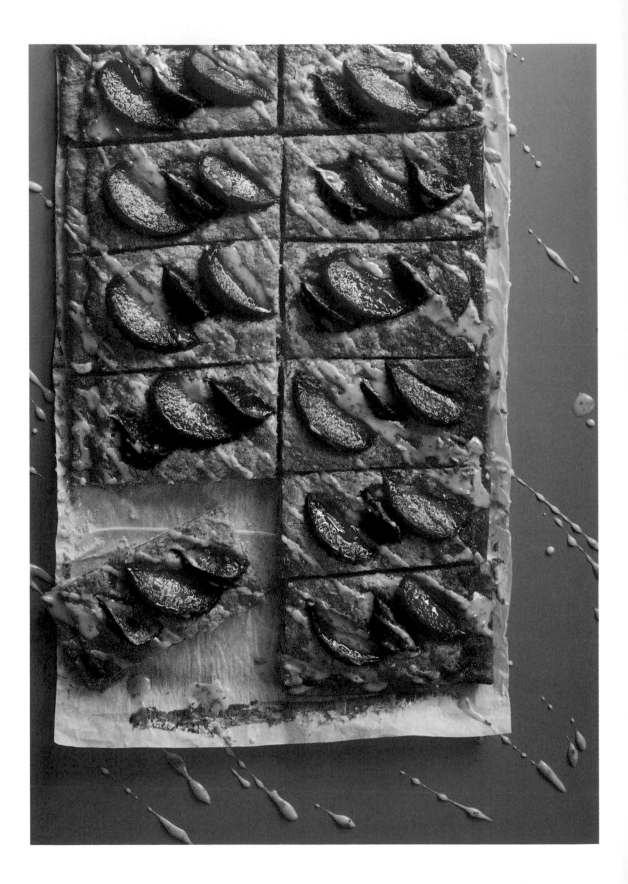

Fruity frangipane fingers

For speed and ease, packs of ready rolled pastry are a lifesaver. Here, I have spread the pastry with some fruity jam and frangipane (a classic sweet almond mixture), and topped it with fruit before baking. This is where you can be very flexible as the fruit can be whatever you like depending on the season, preference or availability. Cut into fingers and drizzled with a tangy icing, these make a nice treat – although you can also cut them into larger portions and serve as a dessert.

320g/11½ oz sheet ready rolled
   shortcrust pastry
100g/3½ oz/½ cup butter, softened
100g/3½ oz/½ cup caster (superfine)
   sugar, plus 2 tbsp, for sprinkling
100g/3½ oz/1 cup ground almonds
finely grated zest of ½ orange or lemon
1 tbsp plain (all-purpose) flour
pinch of flaked sea salt
1 egg, beaten
2 tbsp fruit jam (jelly), try to link
   the flavour with your chosen fruit
your choice of fruit, such as 2–3 pears
   or apples, 4–6 plums or figs, 200g/7 oz
   fresh or frozen berries

For the glaze (optional)
4 tbsp icing (confectioners') sugar
1 tsp lemon or orange juice

Prep 20 minutes / **Cooking** 35 minutes / **Makes** 12 slices

Heat the oven to 200°C/180°C fan/400°F/gas 6.

Unroll the pastry and lay on a parchment-lined baking tray. Using the tip of a sharp knife, score a border 1cm/½ inch from the edge of the pastry. Prick the base all over with a fork. Place in the oven and bake for 10 minutes.

While the pastry is baking, beat together the butter and sugar using electric beaters until light and creamy. Add the ground almonds, orange or lemon zest, flour, salt and egg (reserving a very small amount to brush the pastry edges) and beat until combined.

Gently spread the jam in a thin layer over the top of the pastry, then spread the frangipane on top. Brush the pastry edges with the reserved beaten egg. If you haven't reserved any – don't panic, you can use some melted butter instead.

Depending on the fruit you are using, remove any stones or cores and cut into slices. Arrange on top of the frangipane, in rows so it's easier to cut into fingers when cooked. Sprinkle over the remaining sugar and bake for 25 minutes, or until golden and the frangipane is set.

Once cooked, leave to cool for about 15 minutes, before cutting into fingers. Mix together the icing sugar and just enough orange or lemon juice to give you a thick drizzling consistency. Finish the fruity frangipane fingers by drizzling over the icing and leave to set for 5 minutes or so.

Flexible

Nut-free: *if you can't eat nuts, then this recipe doesn't need to be ruled out. Pine nuts make a great substitute, or if they are off the list, then pumpkin seeds work just as well. Whichever you use, blitz until they resemble ground almonds and use as above, with the addition of an extra 1 tablespoon plain (all-purpose) flour to bind the frangipane.*

Gluten-free: *use a pack of ready rolled gluten-free pastry and use any gluten-free flour in the frangipane. My particular favourite would be buckwheat flour for it's nutty flavour.*

Apricot, pistachio and apple samosas

You'd not usually think of samosas being sweet but there's no reason why they can't be. I've used the traditional method of folding sheets of filo pastry around a filling to form a triangle shape, but rather than deep-frying, these crunchy fruity filo triangles are baked in the oven making them super crisp. Serve as a snack any time of day.

150g/5½ oz dried apricots

1 small–medium cooking apple, peeled

50g/1¾ oz/⅔ cup desiccated (shredded) coconut

75g/2¾ oz pistachio nuts, roughly chopped

finely grated zest and juice of 1 large orange

2 tbsp golden (corn) syrup or maple syrup

½ tsp ground cardamom

½ tsp ground cinnamon

6 sheets filo pastry

4 tbsp coconut oil, melted, or sunflower oil

2 tbsp icing (confectioners') sugar

Prep 30 minutes, plus 1 hour resting / **Cooking** 20 minutes / **Makes** 18

Cut the apricot into small pieces, about 5mm/¼ inch in size and grate the apple. Put the fruit in a bowl along with the desiccated coconut, pistachios, orange zest and juice, syrup and the ground cardamon and cinnamon. Mix well and leave at room temperature for up to 1 hour for all of the flavours to develop together and the dried apricots to soften in the orange.

Heat the oven to 200°C/180°C fan/400°F/gas 6.

Place the filo pastry sheets on the worktop with the short side facing you and with a sharp knife cut the pastry into three vertical strips giving you 18 long pieces in total. Loosely cover with a tea towel to prevent the pastry from drying out.

Working on the top 3 strips at a time, brush each one lightly with oil. Spoon a heaped tablespoon of the filling onto the bottom corner of each lightly oiled pastry strip. Fold over diagonally to create a triangle over the filling. Continue to fold/roll the pastry around the filling, keeping the triangle shape, securing in the filling. Once all 3 strips are filled and folded, sit them on the baking tray. Continue with the remaining strips of pastry until you have used all the filling and pastry strips.

Brush the samosas all over with oil and dust over some icing sugar. Bake for 15–20 minutes until the pastry is golden and crisp.

Once cooked, leave to cool for a few minutes before eating warm, or leave to cool completely and enjoy cold.

Flexible

Flavour swap: *to make an **apple pie** filling, mix together 1 peeled and grated cooking apple and 1 peeled, cored and diced cooking apple, 75g / 2¾ oz / ½ cup sultanas (golden raisins), finely grated zest of ½ lemon, 2 tablespoons golden (corn) syrup, ½ teaspoon mixed (apple pie) spice. Assemble and bake as above.*

*For festive **mince pie samosas**, simply use a jar of mincemeat, mixed with 1 peeled and grated cooking apple for the filling, adding a few chopped almonds if you fancy. Assemble and bake as above.*

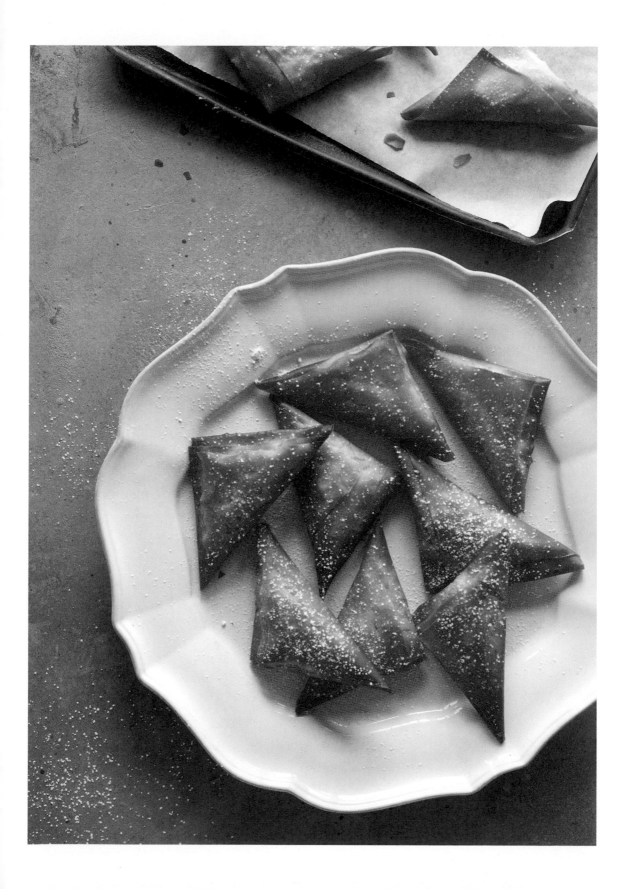

Blueberry crumble pie

with yoghurt pastry

This is bursting with blueberry flavour and possibly one of my favourite pie recipes. Great for enjoying blueberries when they are in season – though frozen blueberries work just as well.. Allow time for this to settle once cooked, rather than diving straight in so the blueberries can thicken and hold their shape in the pie, otherwise you will have a pool of juice on your plate.

I like to use wholemeal flour in the pastry as I think it gives a nice flavour, however a spelt flour or plain white flour will work just as well.

For the pastry
225g/8 oz/1¾ cups plain (all-purpose) wholemeal (wholewheat) flour, plus extra for dusting
1 tbsp caster (superfine) sugar
¼ tsp fine sea salt
125g/4½ oz/½ cup butter, chilled and diced
75g/2¾ oz/⅓ cup natural yoghurt

For the topping
75g/2¾ oz/scant ½ cup porridge (oatmeal) oats
50g/1¾ oz/⅓ cup plain (all-purpose) flour
75g/2¾ oz/⅓ cup soft light brown sugar
1 tsp ground cinnamon
½ tsp flaked sea salt
100g/3½ oz/¾ cup butter, chilled and diced

For the filling
600g/1 lb 5 oz fresh or frozen blueberries
100g/3½ oz/½ cup caster (superfine) sugar
20g/¾ oz cornflour (cornstarch)
1 tbsp lemon juice

Prep 50 minutes, plus 2 hours cooling / **Cooking** 1 hour / **Serves** 8–10

To make the pastry, put the flour, sugar and salt into a large bowl, or food processor. Add the butter and rub or blitz to a fine crumb. Add the yoghurt and bring everything together until you have a smooth dough. If the dough seems a little dry – add a little more yoghurt or a splash of milk.

Roll the pastry on a generously floured surface, so it's big enough to fit inside a 23cm/9 inch pie tin or baking dish. Press into the edges of the dish and leave any excess pastry hanging over. Put in the fridge to rest for about 30 minutes.

Meanwhile, make the crumble topping by simply rubbing everything together with the tips of your fingers creating a rough crumbly texture. Chill in the fridge until ready to use.

In a separate bowl, mix together all of the filling ingredients and set aside.

Heat the oven to 180°C/160°C fan/350°F/gas 4. Put a baking tray in the oven to heat up.

Remove the pastry case from the fridge and trim the excess edges of the pastry. Spoon in the filling, then scatter the crumble on top. Put on the hot baking tray and bake for 1 hour, until the filling is bubbling and the crumble is golden.

Cool for at least 2 hours for the filling to thicken and serve at room temperature.

Flexible

Dairy-free: the pastry can be made using an unsweetened dairy-free yoghurt such as coconut or soya, and make sure you use a plant-based butter in the pastry and crumble.

Gluten-free: be sure to use gluten-free oats and a gluten-free flour blend can be used in both the pastry and crumble. It will be fairly delicate, but any holes can easily be patched up with any trimmings before you add the filling.

*Flavour swap: for a **cherry pie**, the same weight of pitted fresh or frozen cherries can be used instead of blueberries.*

Fig and spelt galette

A galette is an open pie that doesn't require any pressing into a tin or pre-baking, so it is ideal for those wanting a quick and rustic pastry tart. You can fill with whatever fruit you fancy. I love making the most of figs when they're around, and these are baked with some bittersweet orange marmalade that bubbles around the figs making a sticky sauce.

I've used spelt flour in the pastry as it's wholesome nutty flavour is delicious with the figs, although a plain white or wholemeal flour would work equally as well.

For the pastry

175g/6 oz/1⅓ cups spelt flour,
   plus extra for dusting

1 tbsp caster (superfine) sugar

¼ tsp fine sea salt

150g/5½ oz/⅔ cup butter, chilled
   and diced

4–6 tbsp ice cold water

For the filling

4 tbsp orange marmalade

300g/10½ oz fresh ripe figs, quartered

1 egg, beaten, for glazing

3 tbsp demerara (turbinado) sugar

Prep 30 minutes, plus 1 hour chilling / **Cooking** 45 minutes /
Serves 8

To make the pastry, put the flour, sugar and salt into a large bowl, or food processor. Add the butter and rub or blitz to a fine crumb. Add 4 tablespoons ice-cold water and bring everything together until you have a dough, adding the remaining water if required. You should end up with a soft dough consistency.

Tip the pastry out onto a lightly floured worktop and shape into a ball. Flatten to a thick disk, wrap in cling film and put in the fridge for about 1 hour to chill.

Heat the oven to 180°C/160°C fan/350°F/gas 4.

Roll the chilled pastry on a large piece of baking parchment until roughly 3mm/⅛ inch thick, making it into a rough circle.

Spread the marmalade on top of the pastry, leaving a large border of about 3cm/1¼ inch. Scatter the figs on top of the marmalade. Fold the excess pastry up and over the figs, leaving the majority of the figs exposed. Brush the beaten egg over the top of the figs and pastry. Scatter the filling and pastry with demerara sugar and slide a baking tray under the baking parchment.

Bake for 45 minutes until the pastry is golden and the fruit is bubbling. Once out of the oven, leave to cool on the tray for at least 15 minutes.

Serve the galette cut into wedges, warm or cool.

Flexible

Gluten-free: *spelt flour is not gluten-free so a great alternative to keep a slightly nutty flavour would be to use the same quantity of buckwheat flour with the addition of ½ teaspoon xanthan gum. You can also use a standard gluten-free flour blend.*

Vegan: *use a plant-based butter alternative when making the pastry. The pastry can be brushed with 1 teaspoon vegetable oil mixed with 2 teaspoons agave or golden (corn) syrup.*

Flavour swap: *you can be as creative with the fruits and jam (jelly), depending on seasons. Try sliced peaches or nectarines with blueberry jam or sliced apricots with strawberry or raspberry jam.*

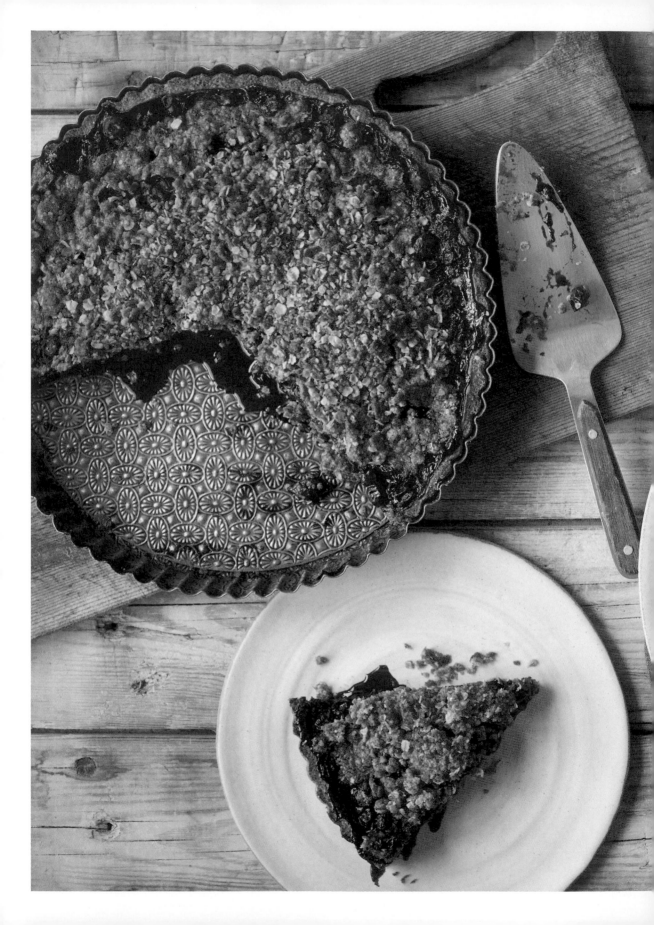

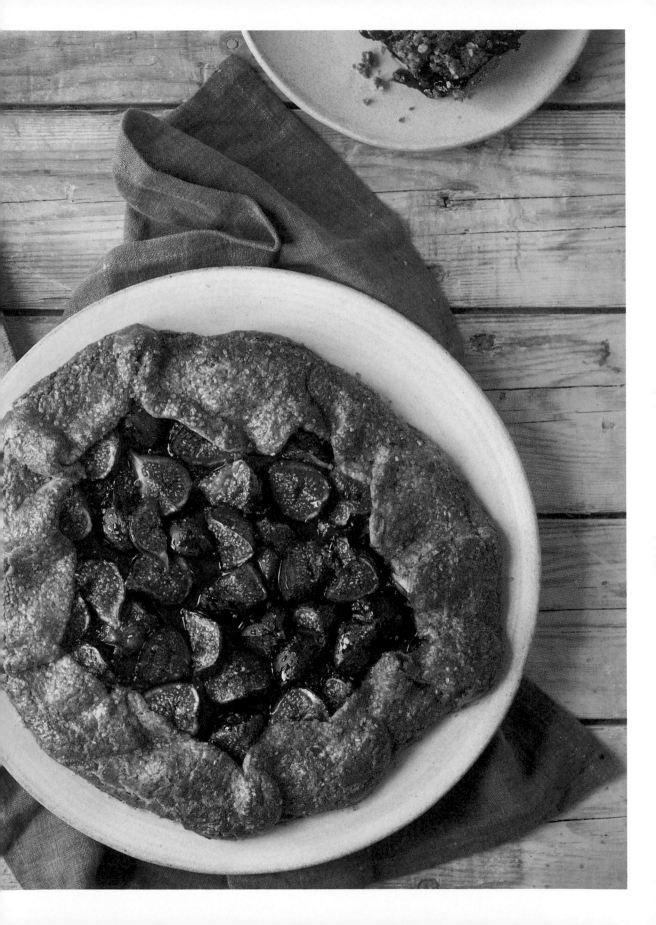

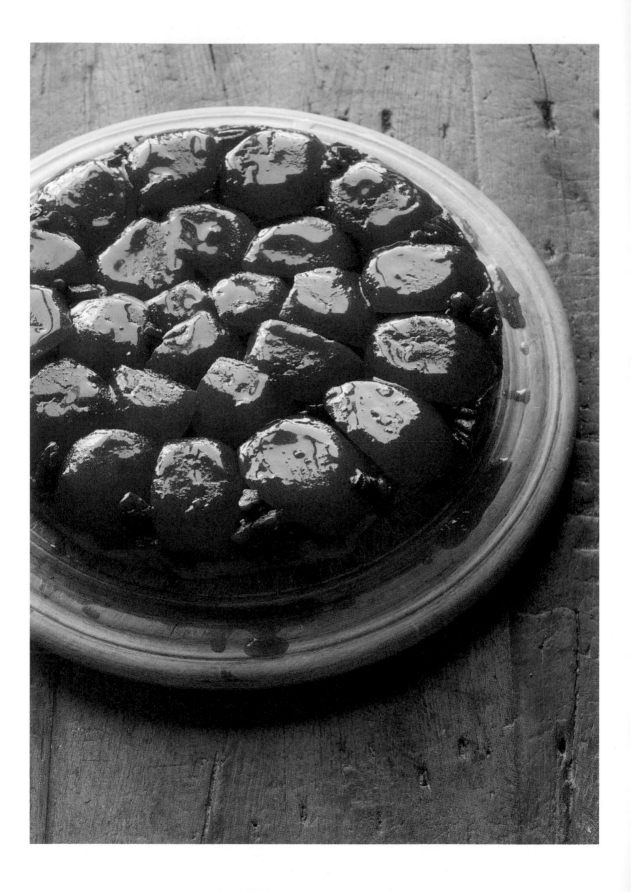

Salted caramel, apple and pecan tarte tatin

This glorious sticky sweet French dessert is hard to resist no matter how full you might be at the end of a meal. I've added some flaked sea salt and pecan nuts to the classic recipe but feel free to omit these if you're a traditionalist.

This is pretty easy to prepare – the oven does all the hard work for you – and can be made a day or two before serving. Keep in the pan in the fridge, then reheat in the oven for 20 mins at 150°C / 130°C fan / 300°F / gas 2 an hour before serving.

320g/11 oz sheet ready rolled puff pastry
900g/2 lb eating apples
25g/1 oz butter, melted

For the caramel
100g/3½ oz/½ cup caster (superfine) sugar
60g/2 oz/¼ cup butter, chilled and diced
50g/1¾ oz/½ cup pecan nuts, roughly chopped
1 tsp flaked sea salt

Prep 20 minutes, plus 30 minutes cooling / **Cooking** 40 minutes / **Serves** 6

Heat the oven to 180°C/160°C fan/350°F/gas 4.

Cut a 23cm/9 inch circle of pastry using a plate as a guide. Prick all over with a fork, sit on the plate and keep cold in the fridge.

Peel, core and quarter the apples and transfer to a large mixing bowl. Drizzle over the melted butter and toss to combine.

Put a 20cm/8 inch ovenproof heavy-based frying pan over a medium-high heat and sprinkle in the sugar. Cook for around 6 minutes, swirling the pan a couple of times (but do not stir) until you have a dark amber caramel colour. Remove from the heat and add the chilled butter and salt, swirling into the pan to create a caramel sauce.

Snugly arrange the apples in the pan cut side up, starting from the outside and working your way into the centre, leaving as few gaps as possible as the apples will shrink when cooking. Take care not to burn your fingers as the caramel will be hot.

Bake for 30 minutes. Have a heatproof mat ready, then remove the pan from the oven (be careful as the handle will be hot). Scatter the pecan nuts over the apples. Place the pastry disk on top. Tuck the edges down the inside of the pan using the back of a spoon, then prick holes in the pastry with a sharp knife to allow any steam to escape.

Bake for a further 40 minutes until the pastry is golden and crisp.

Cool for about 30 minutes before turning out onto a large plate that is big enough to hold any juices that roll off the tart.

Flexible

Vegan: *many shop-bought puff pastries are vegan, although make sure you check the packaging. Any labelled 'all-butter' won't be suitable. As for adapting the rest of the recipe, you'll just need to use a plant-based butter alternative.*

Flavour swap: *to make a **pear and salted honey tart tatin**, replace 50g / 1¾ oz / ¼ cup of the sugar with 50g / 1¾ oz honey and make the caramel as above. Swap the apples for 5–6 small pears, peeled, cored and halved. Arrange snugly in the pan, cut side up and cook as above.*

Passion fruit tart

with coconut pastry

*I really wanted to create a super
tasty, sweet pastry tart that is both
dairy-free and gluten-free, that doesn't
compromise on flavour in any way at
all, and this ticks all of those boxes.
The crisp pastry has just enough
coconut flavour to not be overpowering
and the creamy filling has just the
right amount of passion fruit tartness.*

For the pastry

50g/1¾ oz coconut flour

50g/1¾ oz/½ cup ground almonds,
    plus 1 tbsp for scattering

1 tbsp caster (superfine) sugar

½ tsp fine sea salt

50g/1¾ oz coconut oil, softened
    (use refined coconut oil for a
    more delicate flavour), plus extra
    for greasing

1 egg, beaten

1 tbsp lemon or lime juice

For the filling

150ml/5 fl oz/⅔ cup coconut cream

1 egg and 2 egg yolks

75g/2¾ oz/⅓ cup caster (superfine) sugar

1 tbsp lemon or lime juice

4–5 ripe passion fruit (to make
    100ml/3½ fl oz passion fruit pulp)

toasted coconut flakes, to decorate

Prep 45 minutes / **Cooking** 55 minutes / **Serves** 6–8

Heat the oven to 180°C/160°C fan/350°F/gas 4. Lightly grease a
20cm/8 inch loose-bottomed tart tin with a little coconut oil.

To make the pastry, put the coconut flour, ground almonds, sugar
and salt in a mixing bowl. Add the coconut oil and using a fork,
mash it into the flour until it resembles breadcrumbs. Make a well
in the centre and gradually add the egg and lemon or lime juice and
bring everything together until you have a soft dough (you may not
require all of the egg mixture). Lightly knead and bring to a soft ball
with your hands. Sit on a piece of baking parchment scattered with
some ground almonds and add another piece of parchment on top.
Flatten with the palm of your hand, then leave to rest for 5 minutes.

Roll out the pastry between the parchment, to make a circle big
enough to line the base and sides of the tin. Carefully transfer into
the tin. If it breaks or falls apart just press the pastry into the tin
sealing the cracks with your fingers. It's a very forgiving pastry, and
it's more important to make sure there are no holes. Cut away any
pastry that overhangs the side of the tin and reserve the pastry
trimmings to patch up any holes that may appear once it's cooked.

Sit on a baking tray and bake for 20 minutes until golden and firm
to touch. Reduce the oven to 160°C/140°C/325°F/gas 3.

To make the filling, whisk together the coconut cream, eggs, sugar
and lemon or lime juice in a jug. Keep back 1 tablespoon/15ml of the
passion fruit pulp, and stir the rest into the jug. Pour into the pastry
and bake for 25–35 minutes or until the filling is just set.

Cool to room temperature. Pop in the fridge until needed and serve
cold topped with the reserved passion fruit and toasted coconut.

Flexible

*Dairy swap: you can make this dessert using dairy butter in the pastry instead
of coconut oil, and single (light cream) in the filling rather than coconut cream.
The coconut flavour will be much fainter coming only from the coconut flour.*

*Flavour swap: to make a **lemon tart**, when making the filling, simply
swap the passion fruit and the 1 tablespooon lemon or lime juice for 100ml /
3½ fl oz / scant ½ cup lemon juice. Make as above by whisking the juice into the
rest of the filling ingredients before carefully pouring into the pastry case.*

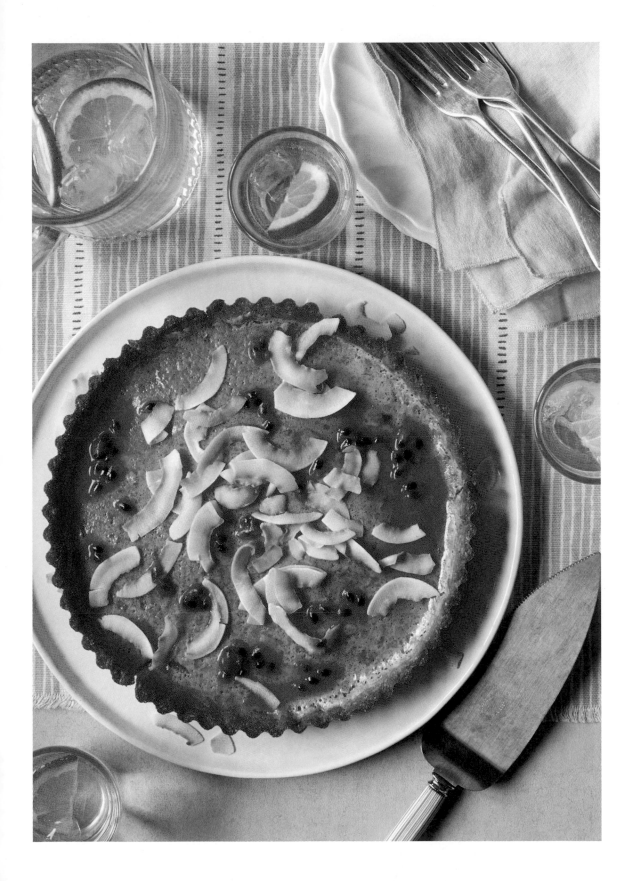

Pecan pumpkin pie

Pecan pie and pumpkin pie are both well-loved, classic recipes, though traditionally neither are suitable for vegan or gluten-free diets. I like a challenge, so have come up with one pie to suit all. My husband Phil wasn't convinced about this working when I explained my idea. He had a slice... and very quickly went back for more, so in my book, that's a winner.

The pastry is made using pecan nuts and has a toffee sweetness from the addition of dates. To top it off there are maple-coated pecan nuts for crunch.

For the pastry
175g/6 oz/1¾ cups pecan nuts
35g/1¼ oz porridge (oatmeal) oats
   (gluten-free)
100g/3½ oz/¾ cup pitted dates
70g/2½ oz coconut oil, melted
½ tsp grated nutmeg
¼ tsp fine sea salt

For the filling
425g/15 oz tinned pumpkin purée
200ml/7 fl oz/generous ¾ cup almond milk
40g/1½ oz/½ cup cornflour (cornstarch)
2 tsp vanilla bean paste
½ tsp ground cinnamon
½ tsp grated nutmeg
3 tbsp maple syrup
100g/3½ oz/½ cup dark brown
   muscovado sugar

For the topping
4 tbsp maple syrup
100g/3½ oz/1 cup pecan nuts

Prep 25 minutes, plus 30 minutes chilling / **Cooking** 65 minutes / **Serves** 8–10

To make the pastry, put the pecans and oats in a food processor and blitz to a fine crumb. Add the dates, coconut oil, nutmeg and a pinch of salt. Blitz really well until you have a thick doughy consistency.

Press the dough into a loose-bottomed 25cm/10 inch tart tin, pushing into the edges and up the sides to evenly line the inside of the tin. Place in the fridge to chill for about 30 minutes.

Heat the oven to 180°C/160°C fan/350°F/gas 4.

Line the pastry case with a piece of baking parchment, making sure the edges of the pastry are loosely covered. Cover the base with baking beans or rice and put in the oven for 15 minutes, then remove the parchment and baking beans. Return the pastry case to the oven and cook for a further 5 minutes until the pastry case is firm and lightly golden.

For the filling, place all the ingredients into a large bowl and whisk together until smooth. Pour the pumpkin mixture into the pastry case and spread into an even layer. Bake for 35 minutes until the filling is starting to set.

For the topping, mix together the pecans and maple syrup, until the nuts are coated. Arrange on top of the pie and return to the oven for a further 10 minutes until golden.

Cool the pie completely in the tin, for a couple of hours at room temperature, before turning out and cutting into wedges to serve.

Flexible

Pumpkin purée: Pumpkin purée is very straightforward to make. You will need a cooking pumpkin (not one that is being sold for carving), around 20cm / 8 inches in diameter. Cut in half and scoop out the seeds and any stringy parts from inside. Place cut side down on a parchment-lined baking tray. Bake at 200°C / 180°C fan / 400°F / gas 6 for around 40–50 minutes until the flesh is really tender when you insert a sharp knife, and it starts to come away from the skin. Once it's cool enough to handle, scoop the flesh from the skin into a blender, and blitz until really smooth (you may need to do this in batches). Cool completely before using or storing in the fridge for up to 1 week.

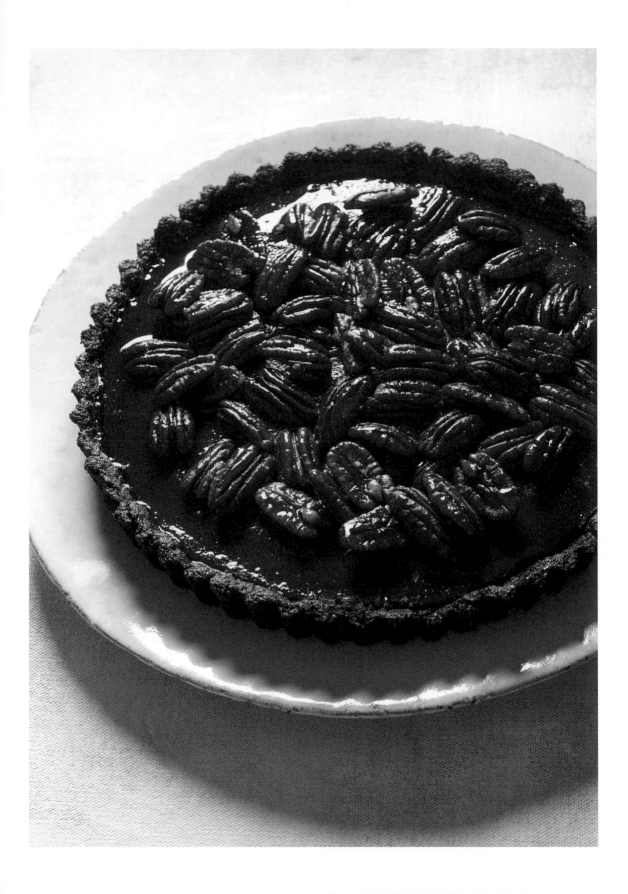

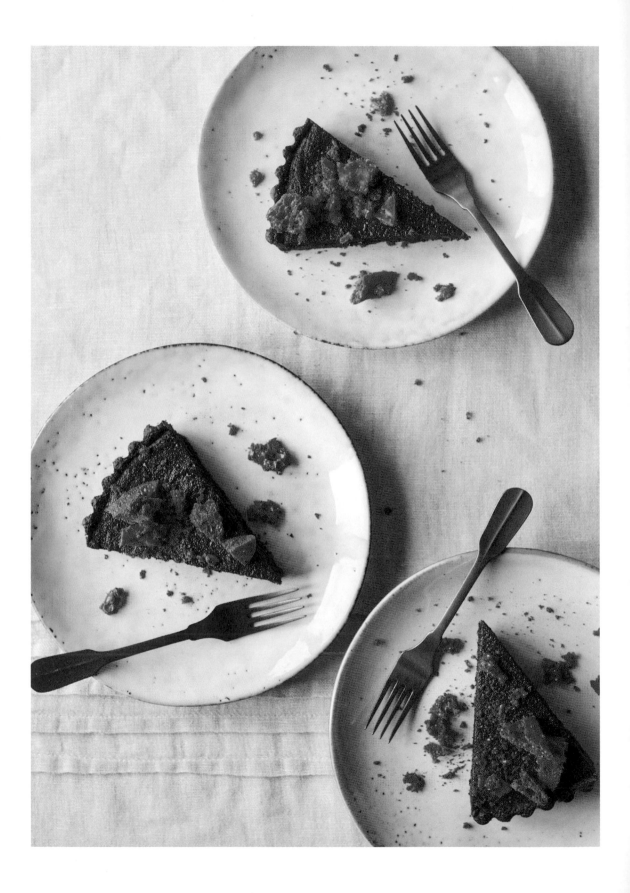

Double chocolate and honeycomb tart

This recipe was written with Rosa, my chocolate-mad daughter, in mind. She, like many people, loves anything chocolatey, so when I first made this tart with its chocolate pastry and rich chocolate filling she was over the moon. To take this from special to another level, her suggestion was to add some honeycomb to the recipe. I think you'll agree it's a very good idea indeed.

For the pastry
125g/4½ oz/1 cup plain (all-purpose) flour, plus extra for dusting
20g/¾ oz cocoa powder
¼ tsp fine sea salt
70g/2½ oz/⅓ cup butter, chilled and diced
2½ tbsp caster (superfine) sugar
2 tbsp milk

For the honeycomb
100g/3½ oz/½ cup caster (superfine) sugar
3 tbsp golden (corn) syrup
1 tsp bicarbonate of (baking) soda

For the filling
200g/7 oz dark chocolate (70 per cent cocoa solids), chopped
150g/5½ oz/⅔ cup butter
1 egg and 3 egg yolks
50g/1¾ oz/¼ cup caster (superfine) sugar
1 tsp vanilla bean paste

Prep 1 hour, plus 1 hour cooling / **Cooking** 32 minutes / **Serves** 8–10

To make the pastry, sift the flour and cocoa powder into a large bowl or food processor and add the salt and butter. Rub or blitz until you have fine breadcrumbs. Add the sugar and milk and bring together into a dough. Wrap in cling film and chill for 30 minutes.

To make the honeycomb, line a small deep heatproof dish or baking tin with baking parchment. Heat the sugar and golden syrup in a saucepan over a low heat. When the sugar has dissolved, increase the heat and simmer until you have an amber-coloured caramel. Immediately stir in the bicarbonate of soda, which will instantly foam. Be careful as it is very hot. Pour straight into the tin and leave for about 1 hour until it sets solid.

Heat the oven to 180°C/160°C fan/350°F/gas 4. Lightly grease a 23cm/9 inch loose-bottomed tart tin.

Dust the worktop with flour and roll out the chilled pastry to line the tin, pressing it into the edges. Trim any excess and line with a piece of baking parchment then pour in some baking beans. Sit on a baking tray and bake for 15 minutes, then remove the parchment and beans, and bake for a further 5 minutes until the pastry is firm.

To make the filling, melt the chocolate and butter in a bowl over a pan of barely simmering water. Alternatively, gently melt in the microwave in 10-second bursts. Whisk together the eggs, sugar and vanilla until you have a very light creamy consistency then fold in the melted chocolate and butter until combined.

Pour the chocolate filling into the pastry case, levelling out the surface, and bake for 12 minutes. The filling will still be wobbly, but as it cools it will firm up a little. Cool to room temperature and transfer to a plate. Crush or break the honeycomb into shards and decorate the top of the tart, serving extra on the side.

Flexible

*Flavour swap: for a **chocolate and raspberry** or **chocolate and cherry tart**, spread 4 tablespoons raspberry or cherry jam (jelly) over the base of the pastry case before pouring over the chocolate filling. Bake as above. Serve with fresh raspberries or cherries and spoonfuls of crème fraîche.*

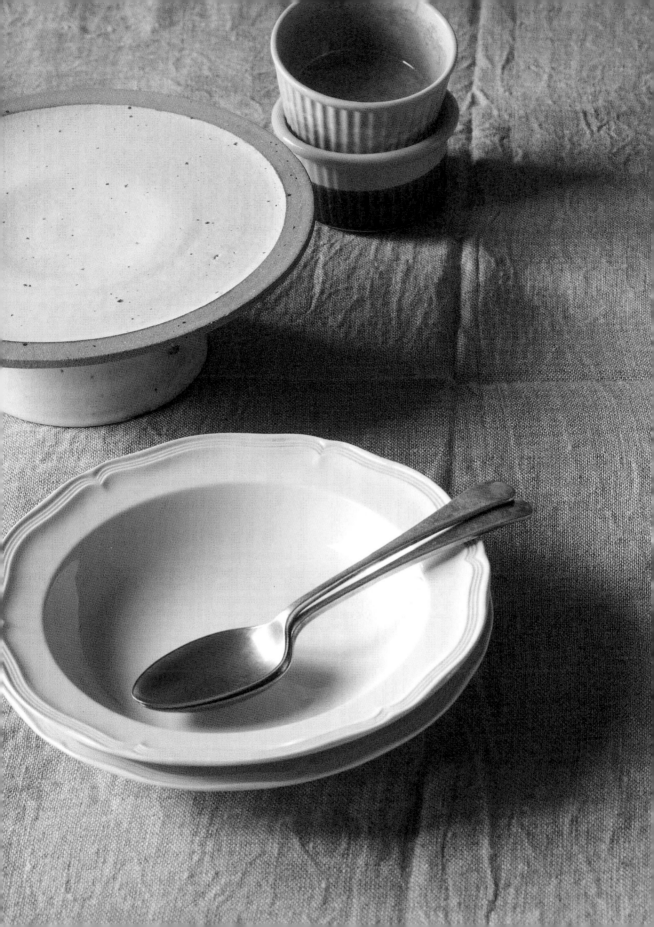

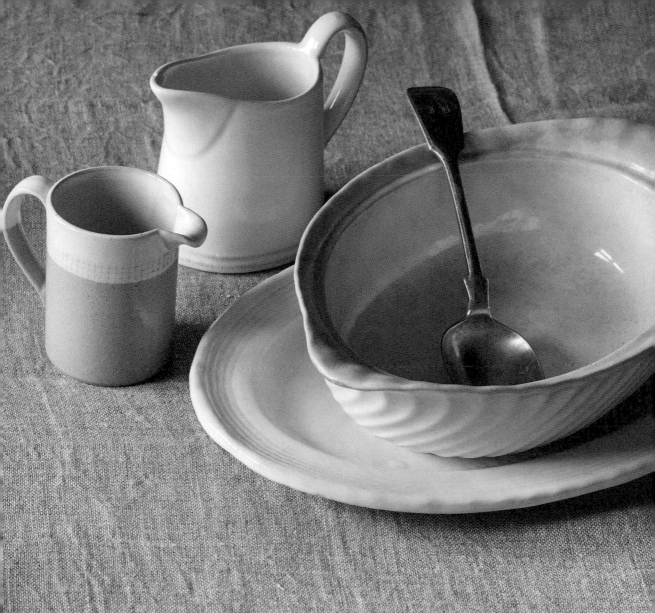

puddings
and desserts

Mint choc chip puddle puddings

Molten chocolate pudding, fondant pudding, melt-in-the-middle chocolate pudding, lava cakes – whatever your preferred name for this pudding, the delightful pool of chocolate sauce when you cut into these desserts is always an impressive end to a meal.

These tasty chocolate and mint puddle puddings are brilliant to serve when entertaining as you can make them in advance and keep chilled for a few days before baking.

115g/4 oz dark chocolate
  (70 per cent cocoa solids), chopped
115g/4 oz/½ cup butter, plus extra
  for greasing
½–¾ tsp peppermint essence
3 eggs and 2 egg yolks
50g/1¾ oz/¼ cup caster (superfine) sugar
50g/1¾ oz/⅓ cup plain (all-purpose) flour
100g/3½ oz white chocolate chips

To serve
cocoa powder, for dusting
white or dark chocolate, to decorate
crème fraîche (optional)

Prep 30 minutes / **Cooking** 10 minutes / **Makes** 6

Heat the oven to 200°C/180°C fan/400°F/gas 6. Grease the insides of six 150ml/5 fl oz ovenproof pudding moulds, coffee cups or ramekins.

Melt the chocolate, butter and peppermint essence in a bowl over a pan of barely simmering water to slowly melt. Alternatively, gently melt in the microwave in 10-second bursts

In a large separate bowl, whisk the eggs and sugar with an electric whisk until they are light, creamy and have doubled in volume. Sift the flour on top, scatter in the white chocolate chips and pour in the buttery chocolate. Fold together taking care not to knock out too much air by overmixing.

Divide the mixture between the moulds, cups or ramekins and sit on a baking tray. Bake for 10 minutes to serve straight away. Or you can keep them covered in the fridge for 2–3 days and cook them when required. Simply make sure you return them to room temperature before cooking.

To serve, turn the hot puddings upside down onto plates and dust with cocoa powder. Grate or shave (using a vegetable peeler) a little white or dark chocolate over the top of each one. Serve straight away alongside a big spoon of crème fraiche if you wish, and when you cut into the middle of each pudding the centre should be soft and molten.

Flexible

Gluten-free: a gluten-free flour blend can be used, or you could also use 50g / 1¾ oz / ½ cup ground almonds, coconut or rice flour.

Dairy-free: make sure you use a dairy-free dark chocolate and omit the white chocolate chips (or use dairy-free dark chocolate chips instead) and use a plant-based butter alternative.

*Flavour swap: for **chocolate orange puddle puddings**, swap the peppermint essence for the finely grated zest of 1 orange and omit the white chocolate chips.*

*For **Turkish delight puddle puddings**, swap the peppermint essence for ½–1 teaspoon rosewater and scatter the finished puddings with roughly chopped pistachio nuts.*

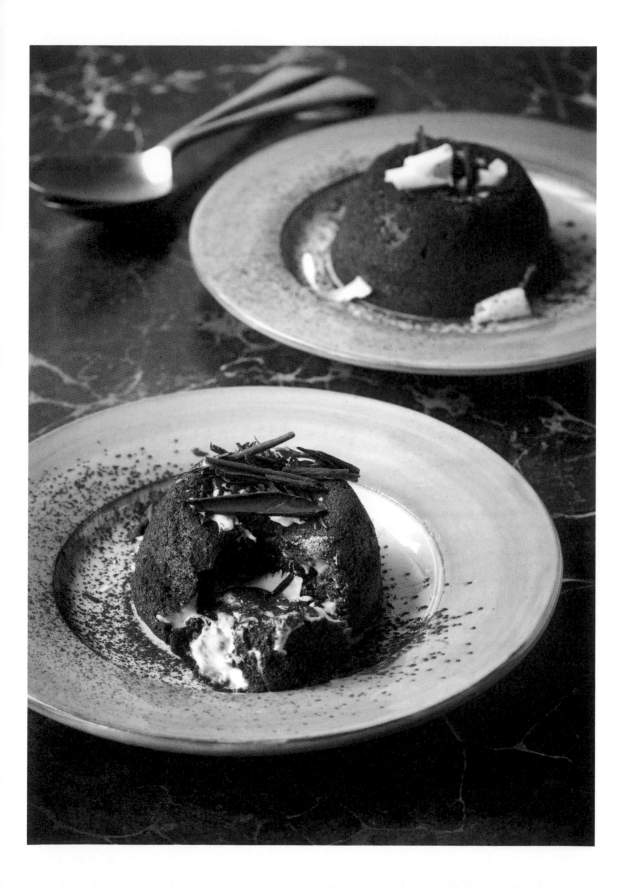

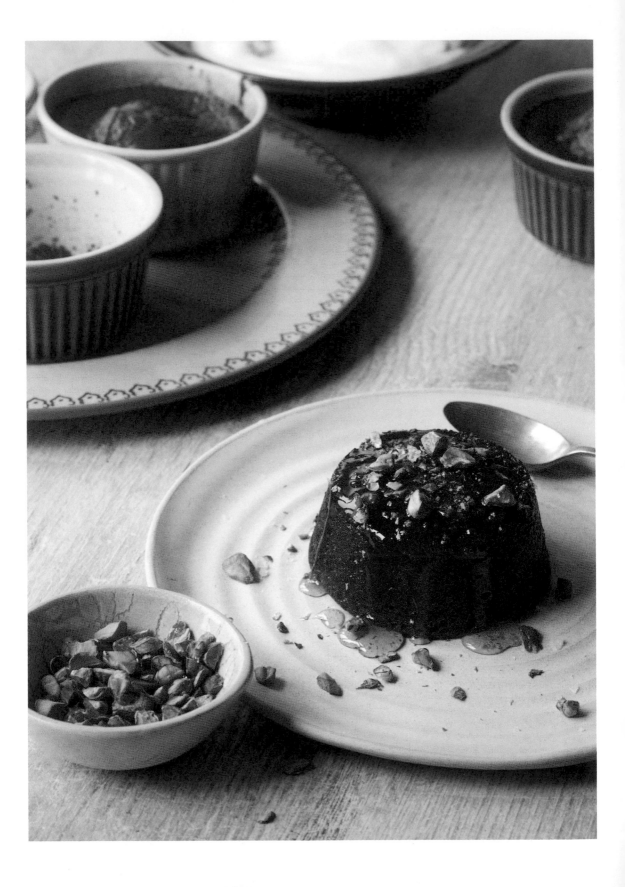

Salted honey and pistachio puddings

*These individual golden puddings
are quick and easy enough to make
as a weekday pudding, yet impressive
enough to serve at the end of a fancy
dinner with hot, salted honey drizzled
over the top, a scattering of green
pistachios and spoonful of Greek
yoghurt on the side. They are light in
texture, full of flavour and brimming
with flexible options for dietary
requirements.*

60g/2 oz honey

100g/3½ oz pistachio nuts,
   plus extra to serve

100g/3½ oz/¾ cup self-raising (self-rising)
   flour

100g/3½ oz/ ½ cup soft light brown sugar

½ tsp bicarbonate of (baking) soda

50g/1¾ oz/⅓ cup butter, melted,
   plus extra for greasing

2 eggs, beaten

175g/6 oz/generous ¾ cup Greek yoghurt,
   plus extra to serve

½ tsp orange blossom water

½ tsp flaked sea salt

Prep 30 minutes / **Cooking** 20 minutes / **Makes** 6

Heat the oven to 180°C/160°C fan/350°F/gas 4. Grease the insides of
six 200ml/7 fl oz ovenproof pudding moulds, coffee cups or ramekins,
and line the bases with a small circle of baking parchment. Add
1 teaspoon honey into the bottom of each one.

Put the pistachios in a food processor and blitz until they are finely
ground. Mix in the flour, sugar and bicarbonate of soda. Add the
melted butter, eggs, yoghurt and orange blossom water and briefly
blitz to combine.

Transfer to the buttered moulds, level the surface with the back of a
spoon and sit on a baking tray. Bake for 20 minutes until golden and
risen, and a skewer comes out clean when inserted in the centre.

Put the remaining honey in a small saucepan over a medium-high
heat. When it starts to bubble, stir in the salt and remove from
the heat.

Loosen the edge of each pudding with a round-bladed knife and turn
out onto plates. Remove the parchment disk, and spoon over the hot
salted honey. Scatter over pistachios and serve hot with a dollop of
Greek yoghurt.

Flexible

Vegan: *first of all, you will need to use the same weight of maple
syrup instead of honey and use it in the same way as above. Swap
the butter and yoghurt for plant-based alternatives, and instead
of eggs, mix together 2 tablespoons chia seeds with 6 tablespoons
cold water, leave to thicken for 10 minutes and use as you would
the eggs.*

Flavour swap: *other nuts can be used in these puddings. Pecan
nuts and walnuts are particularly tasty with the orange blossom
water, which you can always swap for finely grated orange zest
should you prefer. Maple syrup can be used instead of honey for a
milder flavour.*

Chocolate, cherry and mascarpone torte

A chocolate dessert will always go down well and this has a retro touch to it too. The combination of chocolate, cherries and cream are the wonderful ingredients making up the well-loved Black Forest gateau. It was hugely popular in the 1970s, and a cake my sister Millie and I would have eaten for breakfast, lunch and dinner given half a chance when growing up!

Serve warm with ice cream, cream or crème fraîche and a glass of chilled kirsch (cherry liqueur) for a real treat. Any leftover torte is just as delicious over the next couple of days served cold.

125g/4½ oz/½ cup butter

50g/1¾ oz/½ cup cocoa powder, plus extra for dusting

75g/2¾ oz cherry jam (jelly)

150g/5½ oz/¾ cup caster (superfine) sugar

2 eggs and 1 egg yolk

100g/3½ oz/1 cup ground almonds

1 tsp baking powder (gluten-free)

100g/3½ oz/½ cup mascarpone cheese

150g/5½ oz fresh, frozen (and defrosted) or tinned cherries, pitted

ice cream, crème fraîche or pouring cream (with an added splash of kirsch for a boozy kick, if you like), to serve

Prep 35 minutes / **Cooking** 25 minutes / **Serves** 8

Heat the oven to 180°C/160°C fan/350°F/gas 4. Grease a 24cm/ 9½ inch loose-bottomed tart tin.

Melt the butter in a medium saucepan, over a low heat and then sift in the cocoa powder. Stir until the mixture starts to bubble and then remove from the heat. Add the jam, 100g/3½ oz/½ cup of the sugar, the whole eggs (not the separate yolk), ground almonds and baking powder. Pour into the tin and keep to one side.

Mix together the mascarpone, egg yolk, remaining sugar and place spoonfuls on top of the chocolate mixture. Pull a knife backwards and forwards a few times to create a marbled effect. Scatter over the cherries and press down lightly to partially cover in the mixture.

Put the tin on a baking tray and bake for 25 minutes until the torte has risen slightly and is just firm to touch.

Leave to cool slightly before removing from the tin, dust with cocoa powder, if liked, and serve warm, or leave to cool completely in the tin. Serve with ice cream, crème fraîche or pouring cream.

Flexible

Nut-free: *the ground almonds can be swapped for the same weight of plain (all-purpose) flour or a gluten-free flour blend is also fine if necessary.*

Dairy-free: *use a plant-based butter and swap the mascarpone for a plant-based alternative. If you can't find a suitable mascarpone, then a low-fat cream cheese alternative would work just as well.*

Flavour swap: *raspberry jam (jelly) and fresh or frozen raspberries can be used instead of cherries. A grating of orange zest is also a nice addition with raspberries.*

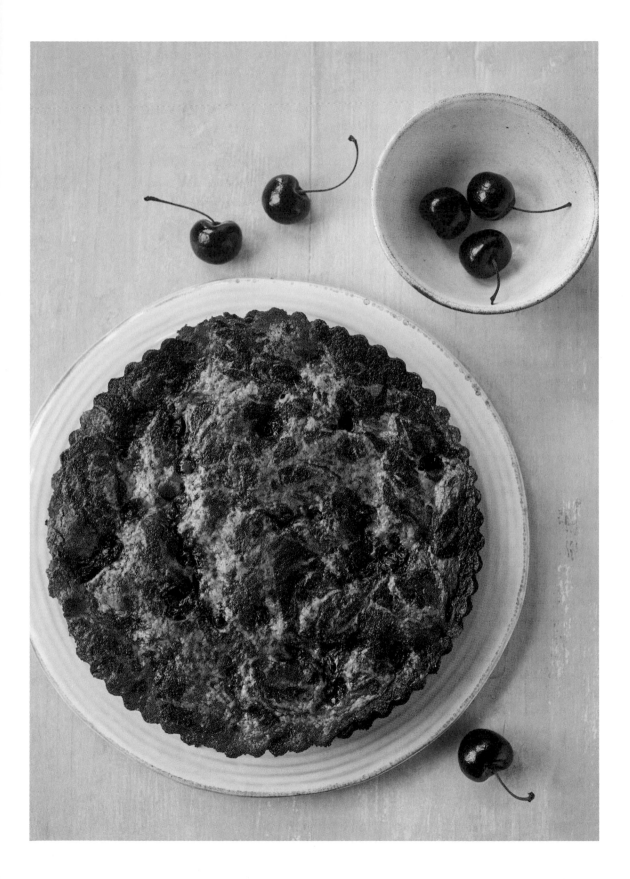

Baked blueberry cheesecake

It's hard not to go over-board when describing this recipe, but it really is absolutely delicious and as one of my lovely friends Jules said to me when I gave him a huge slice to try, it was the best cheesecake he has ever eaten! The light yet rich creamy cheesecake filling is studded with pops of blueberries, which is encased in crunchy biscuit crumb and to top things off there are even more juicy, glossy blueberries spooned over the top. This is a dessert not to be rushed, but with a little patience you'll be more than impressed with the end result.

For the base

200g/7 oz digestive biscuits
   (Graham Crackers)
100g/3½ oz/½ cup butter, melted

For the filling

500g/1 lb 2 oz/2⅓ cups full fat cream
   cheese
250g/9 oz/1¼ cups caster (superfine)
   sugar
2 tbsp cornflour (cornstarch)
2 tsp vanilla bean paste
125ml/4 fl oz/½ cup soured cream
3 eggs, beaten
250g/9 oz/2 cups fresh or frozen
   blueberries

For the topping

250g/9 oz/2 cups fresh or frozen
   blueberries
60g/2 oz/¼ cup caster (superfine)
   sugar
2 tbsp lemon juice
1 tsp cornflour (cornstarch)

Prep 40 minutes, plus 6 hours (or overnight) cooling and chilling /
Cooking 1 hour / **Serves** 10–12

Heat the oven to 160°C/140°C fan/325°F/gas 3. Grease a 20cm/
8 inch springform cake tin, and line with baking parchment.

Place the biscuits in a plastic bag and crush with a rolling pin to fine crumbs. Pour the melted butter into the biscuits and mix until combined. Press the biscuits into the base and up the sides of the tin to create an even layer. Chill in the fridge for 20 minutes to set.

In a large bowl, beat together the cream cheese, sugar, cornflour and vanilla until smooth. Add the soured cream and briefly beat again, avoiding adding too much air as this will cause the filling to crack when cooking. Gradually add the eggs, beating until smooth.

Stir in the blueberries and pour onto the base. Sit on a baking tray and cook for 1 hour until the top is lightly golden, a little puffed up, and has a slight wobble when you give the tray a shake. Leave for a few minutes more if you feel it's not quite there.

Once cooked, turn off the oven and prop open the door so that it is ajar. Leave the cheesecake to cool in the oven for about 2 hours. Once the oven is cool, transfer the cheesecake to the fridge to chill for at least 4 hours or overnight.

Put half of the blueberries for the topping in a small saucepan with the sugar and 1 tablespoon lemon juice. Simmer for 5 minutes until the blueberries break down. Whisk the remaining lemon juice into the cornflour, and stir the mixture into the saucepan, with the remaining blueberries. Cook for 1 minute, then remove from the heat and leave to cool and thicken slightly. When ready to serve, spoon the blueberries over the cheesecake.

Flexible

Vegan: for the base, use vegan biscuits and a plant-based butter. For the filling, soak 150g/5½ oz/1¼ cups cashew nuts in cold water overnight to soften. Drain and put in a food processor with 300g/10½ oz silken tofu, 200ml/7 fl oz maple or agave syrup, 100ml/3½ fl oz/scant ½ cup lemon juice, 2 tablespoons cornflour (cornstarch) and 2 teaspoons vanilla bean paste. Blend the mixture well so you have a super smooth batter. Stir in the blueberries, pour onto the base and bake as above for 1 hour. Cool in the oven then refrigerate for a couple of hours then add the topping.

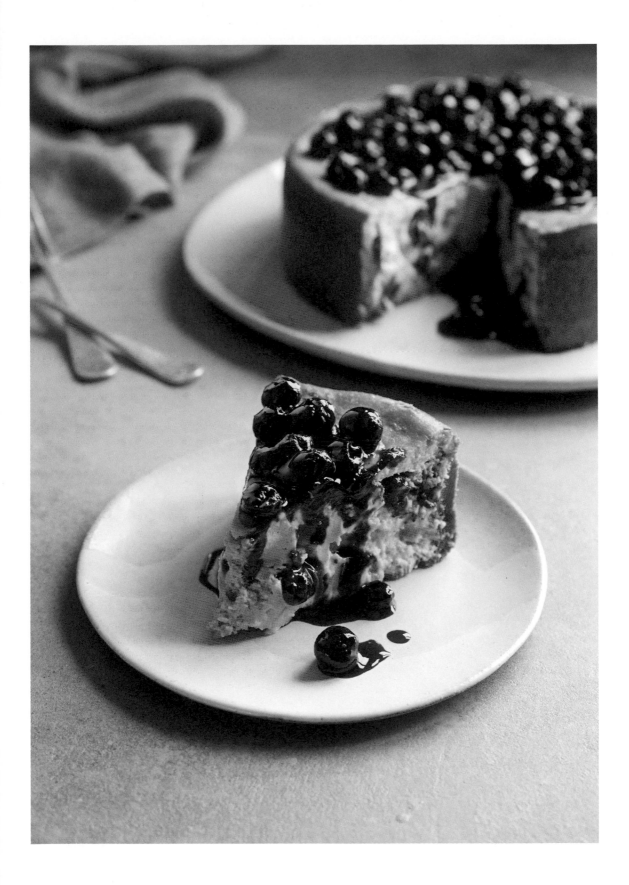

Grapefruit and brown sugar meringue pie

This takes the classic lemon meringue pie to another level. Swapping the lemon filling for beautiful ruby or pink grapefruit makes it mouthwateringly good and a stunning pink colour. As for the meringue topping, I've swapped the usual white sugar for soft brown sugar, which creates a delicate caramel flavour and pairs beautifully with the grapefruit filling.

For the pastry

150g/5½ oz/generous 1 cup plain (all-purpose) flour, plus extra for dusting

1 tbsp caster (superfine) sugar

¼ tsp fine sea salt

100g/3½ oz/½ cup butter, chilled and diced

For the filling

4 large ruby or pink grapefruit

100g/3½ oz/1 cup cornflour (cornstarch)

200g/7 oz/1 cup caster (superfine) sugar

4 egg yolks

25g/1 oz butter, softened

For the meringue

4 egg whites

150g/5½ oz/¾ cup soft brown sugar

2 tsp cornflour (cornstarch)

1 tsp lemon juice

Prep 1 hour, plus 30 minutes chilling / **Cooking** 30–35 minutes / **Serves** 8–10

To make the pastry, put the flour, sugar, butter and salt in a food processor and blitz until it resembles fine breadcrumbs. Alternatively, mix or rub the butter into the dry ingredients to get the same texture. Add 1–2 tablespoons cold water and briefly mix until everything comes together. Knead lightly on a floured worktop until you have a smooth dough. Wrap in cling film and chill in the fridge for 30 minutes.

Heat the oven to 200°C/180°C fan/400°F/gas 6.

Roll out the chilled pastry on a lightly floured surface and use to line a 23cm/9 inch tin, about 3cm/1¼ inches deep. Trim any over-hanging pastry and prick the base several times with a fork. Line the tin with baking parchment, then add some baking beans. Sit on a baking tray and bake for 15 minutes. Remove the parchment and beans and continue to cook for a further 10 minutes until the pastry is lightly golden.

Meanwhile, to make the filling, finely grate the zest from just one of the grapefruit and put into a medium saucepan along with the cornflour and sugar. Squeeze the juice from all of the grapefruit into a measuring jug. You need 700ml/24 fl oz/2¾ cups in total so if it's not quite there, top up with a little water. Pour into the saucepan, stirring until the cornflour dissolves. Place the pan over a medium heat and bring to the boil, stirring all the time until thickened. Simmer for 1 minute, then remove from the heat. Leave to cool for 5 minutes, then briskly beat in the egg yolks and butter. Strain into a bowl then pour into the pastry case.

Reduce the oven to 160°C/140°C fan/325°F/gas 3.

To make the meringue, whisk the egg whites in a large bowl using an electric mixer until you have stiff peaks. Mix together the sugar and cornflour, pinching away any lumps of sugar between your fingertips. Gradually add this and the lemon juice to the eggs, whisking all the time until you have a firm glossy light brown meringue.

Spoon the meringue onto the pie filling, creating swirly peaks with the back of your spoon or by using a palette knife. Bake for about 30–35 minutes until the meringue is golden and crisp.

Cool to room temperature before serving. This is best eaten on the day it's made.

Flexible

Gluten-free: you can use a gluten-free flour blend or, for a slightly different flavour, you could use the recipe for coconut pastry, used in the passion fruit tart on page 154.

Flavour swap: a combination of grapefruit, orange and lime in the filling is delicious – simply squeeze the juice from 2 grapefruit, 1 lime and 2 oranges giving you 750ml / 25 fl oz / 3¼ cups of mixed juice. Use this along with the grated zest from the lime to make the filling as above.

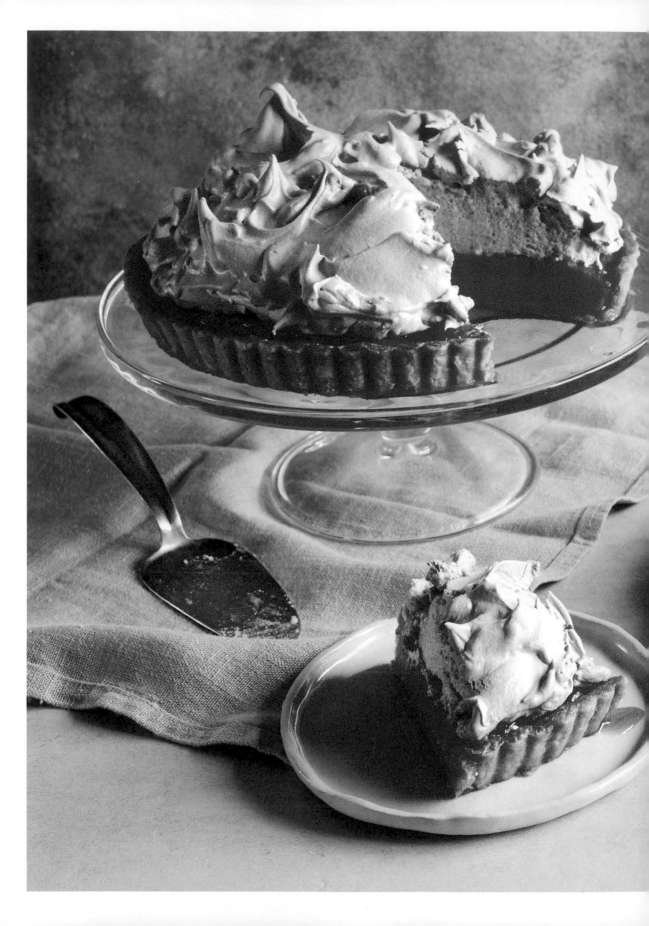

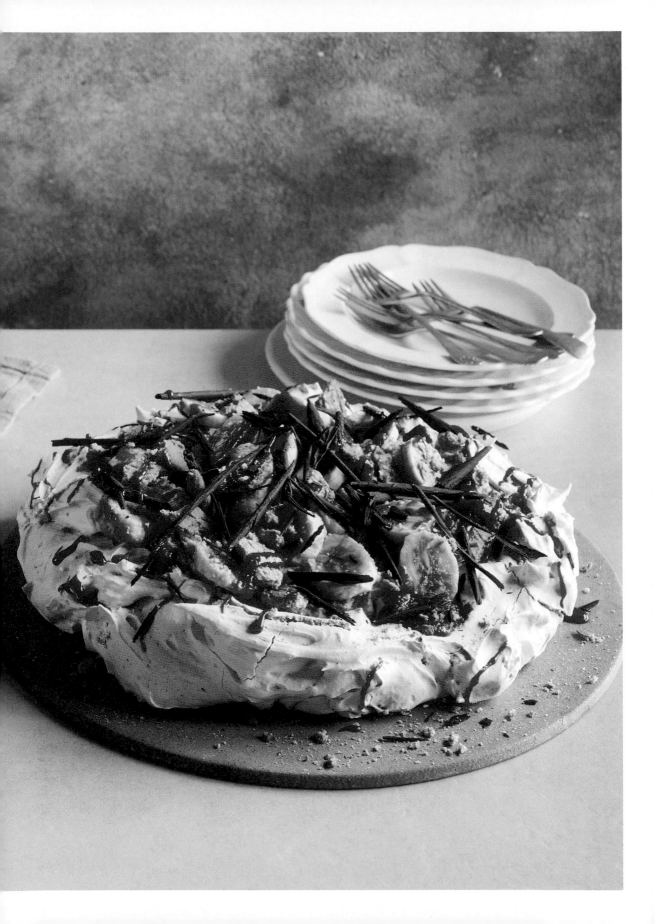

Banoffee pavlova

Oh, hello! When a banoffee pie meets a pavlova (my two all-time favourite desserts), you get the most unbelievable and irresistible end result. Crisp meringue speckled with crushed digestive biscuits, rich banana-flavoured caramel, fluffy cream, more bananas, more crushed digestives, chocolate shavings and more banana caramel. Heavenly.

For the meringue

4 egg whites

225g/8 oz/generous 1 cup caster
   (superfine) sugar

1 tsp cornflour (cornstarch)

1 tsp lemon juice

150g/5½ oz digestive biscuits
   (Graham Crackers), coarsely crumbled

For the caramel

1 medium–large banana

4 tbsp double (heavy) cream

2 tsp vanilla bean paste

200g/7 oz/1 cup caster (superfine) sugar

For the filling

200ml/7 fl oz/generous ¾ cup double
   (heavy) cream

2 bananas, sliced

2 tbsp dark chocolate shavings,
   to decorate

Prep 45 minutes, plus 4 hours (or overnight) cooling /
Cooking 1 hour / **Serves** 8

Heat the oven to 150°C/130°C fan/300°F/gas 2. Draw a 23cm/ 9 inch circle as a template on a sheet of baking parchment and place upside down on a large baking tray.

To make the meringue, whisk the egg whites to stiff peaks in a large bowl using an electric whisk. Mix together the sugar and cornflour, and then gradually whisk into the egg whites along with the lemon juice. Continue to whisk for a few minutes until you have a very stiff glossy meringue. Gently stir in two-thirds of the biscuit crumbs, reserving the rest for serving.

Spoon the meringue onto the baking tray to fill the circle template, creating a dip in the middle and higher sides. Bake for 1 hour, then leave in the oven with the door shut for around 4 hours or overnight, until the meringue is completely cool.

To make the banana caramel, blitz the banana in a food processor until smooth, then mix in the cream and vanilla. Put the sugar and 100ml/3½ fl oz water in a heavy-based pan. Place over a medium heat and stir until the sugar has dissolved. Increase the heat and allow the sugar to become a golden caramel colour, without stirring but swirling the pan a couple of times for even colouring. Remove from the heat and stir in the banana purée, taking care as it will spit and bubble. Once it's smooth, transfer to a heatproof bowl to cool completely.

When ready to serve, whisk the cream until it just starts to form soft peaks. Fold through three-quarters of the banana caramel and spoon into the centre of the pavlova. Arrange the slices of banana on top, drizzle with the remaining banana caramel and finish by scattering over the chocolate shavings and reserved digestive biscuit crumbs.

Flexible

Vegan pavlova: *you can transform this into a vegan recipe with a few changes:*

For the meringue, strain the liquid (aquafaba) from a 400g / 14 oz can of chickpeas and chill in the fridge overnight. Whisk the chilled aquafaba with an electric whisk for around 8 minutes until soft peaks form. Gradually whisk in 200g / 7 oz caster (superfine) sugar mixed with 1 tablespoon cornflour (cornstarch) and 1 teaspoon lemon juice. Whisk for 8 minutes or so until the meringue is thick and glossy. Stir in two-thirds of the biscuit crumbs. Spoon onto the prepared baking tray and put in a preheated oven at 150°C / 130°C fan / 300°F / gas 2. As soon as it goes in the oven reduce the temperature to 130°C / 110°C fan / 260°F / gas ½ and cook for 1¼ hours. Turn off the heat and leave in the oven until completely cool (around 4 hours or overnight).

For the banana caramel, simply use a plant-based cream instead.

For the filling, I really like to use coconut cream as the flavour works well with the banana and caramel. Chill 2 x 400g / 14 oz tins coconut milk in the fridge overnight. When ready, carefully scoop the solid coconut cream from the top of the tins into a large mixing bowl (keeping the liquid for another recipe). Using an electric whisk, whisk the coconut cream until it is light and airy, whisking in 1 tablespoon cornflour (cornstarch) at the end to help stabilize the cream. Continue with the recipe as above.

Tropical meringue roulade

No matter how full you might be at the end of a meal, no one will be able to turn down a slice of this fruity dessert. The pillowy marshmallow meringue is balanced perfectly with the tangy tropical fruits and mellow coconut liqueur.

If you are planning on making this a few hours ahead of serving, then I suggest you firmly wrap the roulade in some baking parchment and chill in the fridge, so it retains its shape.

For the meringue

4 egg whites

175g/6 oz/scant 1 cup caster (superfine) sugar

1 tsp cornflour (cornstarch)

1 tsp lime juice

finely grated zest of 1 lime

icing (confectioners') sugar, for dusting

For the filling

1 ripe mango, peeled and roughly chopped

2 tbsp coconut liqueur

juice of ½ lime

3 tbsp caster (superfine) sugar

200ml/7 fl oz/generous ¾ cup double (heavy) cream

3 ripe passion fruit

To serve

icing (confectioners') sugar, for dusting

handful toasted coconut flakes

finely grated zest of ½ lime

Prep 35 minutes / **Cooking** 25 minutes / **Serves** 6–8

Heat the oven to 180°C/160°C fan/350°F/gas 4. Line a 35 x 25cm x 2cm/14 x 10 x ¾ inch rectangular tin with baking parchment. Line a wire rack with baking parchment and dust with icing sugar.

To make the meringue, whisk the egg whites in a large bowl with an electric mixer until they form soft peaks. Add half of the sugar and continue to whisk for a couple of minutes. Mix the cornflour into the remaining sugar and add to the egg whites with the lime juice and zest. Continue to whisk until you have a firm glossy meringue that holds in stiff peaks.

Spread the meringue over the prepared baking tray. Bake for 25 minutes until lightly browned and just firm to the touch, but not at all solid. The meringue will have puffed up quite a lot but don't worry, it will flatten when cooling. Remove from the oven and immediately turn it out onto the prepared wire rack. Peel away the parchment on the top, and leave the meringue to completely cool.

Put the mango, coconut liqueur, lime juice and sugar in a food processor and blitz to a purée. Whisk the cream until it forms soft peaks, then fold through the mango purée and passion fruit pulp.

Spread the filling onto the meringue, leaving a 2cm/¾ inch border. Starting at one long edge of the meringue, gently roll the roulade away from you into a log shape, ending with the seam underneath. Don't worry if the meringue cracks, this all adds character!

Transfer to a serving plate, dust with more icing sugar, scatter over toasted coconut flakes and a grating of lime zest.

Flexible

Dairy-free: Coconut cream makes a great alternative. Put 2 x 400g / 14 oz tins coconut milk in the fridge and leave overnight. When ready, carefully scoop the solid coconut cream from the top of the cans into a large mixing bowl. Using an electric whisk, whisk the coconut cream until it's light and airy. Whisk in 2 tablespoons icing (confectioners') sugar and 1 tablespoon cornflour (cornstarch). Spread over the meringue roulade and top with the fruit. The coconut cream texture isn't as stable as a dairy cream, so best to make it and assemble just before serving.

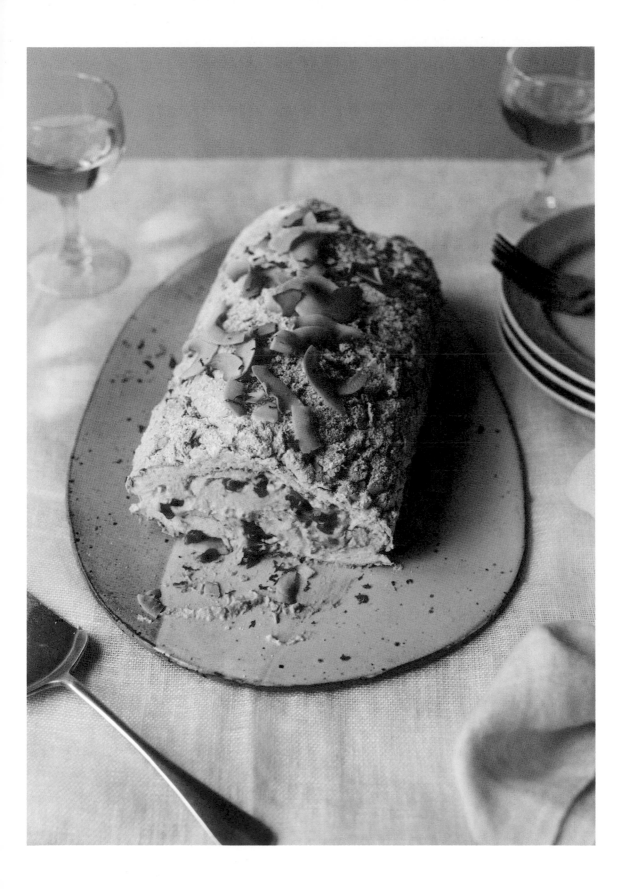

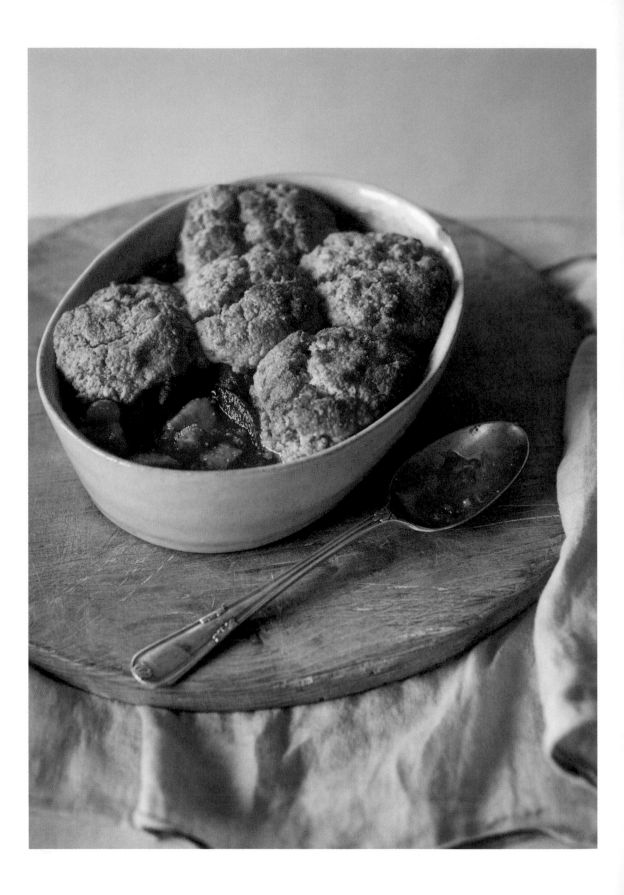

Flexible fruit cobbler

A fruit cobbler has the same comfort food feel to it as a pie or crumble. Your chosen fruit is topped with a scone-like topping that has a crisp crust and soft base from soaking up the fruit juices.

The flexibility of this recipe comes from the type of fruit you use – it's entirely up to you, depending on seasons, preference or availability. The cobbler topping is slightly different from a classic flour mix, as it's made with a blend of naturally gluten-free ingredients and can easily be adapted for vegan or nut-free diets.

For the filling
675–800g/1½ lb–1 lb 12 oz prepared raw
   fruit (I like diced rhubarb, raspberries,
   blackberries, strawberries, diced, peeled
   apple or pear, gooseberries, sliced
   plums, apricots or peaches)
100g/3½ oz/½ cup caster (superfine) sugar
2 tbsp cornflour (cornstarch)
juice of ½ orange

For the topping
85g/3 oz/⅔ cups porridge (oatmeal) oats
   (gluten-free)
85g/3 oz/scant 1 cup ground almonds
85g/3 oz/scant 1 cup rice flour or
   cornflour (cornstarch)
100g/3½ oz/½ cup caster (superfine) sugar
2 tsp baking powder (gluten-free)
¼ tsp flaked sea salt
125g/4½ oz/½ cup butter, chilled and diced
finely grated zest of 1 orange (optional)
1 tsp poppy seeds (optional)
125ml/4 fl oz/½ cup buttermilk or
   natural yoghurt

Prep 25 minutes / **Cooking** 45–55 minutes / **Serves** 6

Heat the oven to 180°C/160°C fan/350°F/gas 4.

Put the prepared fruit in a suitably sized baking dish, it should fill the dish roughly halfway or three-quarters full, leaving a good 2.5cm/1 inch or so of extra space for the cobbler topping. Gently mix in the sugar, cornflour and orange juice. Set aside.

To make the cobbler topping, put the oats in a food processor and blitz until you have a fine powder that resembles flour. Transfer to a large mixing bowl and mix in the ground almonds, rice flour or cornflour, sugar, baking powder and salt. Add the butter and rub in with your fingers until you have a breadcrumb consistency. If you are using the orange zest and poppy seeds, stir them in, then add the buttermilk or yoghurt. Bring the mixture together with a round-ended knife to start with, then use a spoon, until you have a soft, fairly wet dough.

Scoop the cobbler dough in large spoonfuls on top of the filling, being as rustic or neat as you like, leaving plenty of the filling exposed still.

Put on a baking tray and bake for 45–55 minutes until the cobbler is golden and the filling is bubbling around the edges. Cool for at least 20 minutes before serving and enjoy over the next few days hot or cold.

Flexible
Vegan: use a plant-based butter or coconut oil in the topping, and either a plant-based yoghurt (coconut is particularly tasty) or, for a vegan buttermilk, stir 1 teaspoon lemon juice into a plant-based milk such as almond, soya or oat. Sit for 5 minutes to thicken slightly before using.

Nut-free: you can swap the ground almonds and rice flour for 160g/5¾ oz/scant 1¼ cups plain (all-purpose) flour, or a gluten-free flour blend if required.

dietary index

When recipe title is in italics, please refer to the Flexible section on that page.

DAIRY-FREE

GLUTEN-FREE

NUT-FREE + SESAME-FREE

EGG-FREE

recipe index

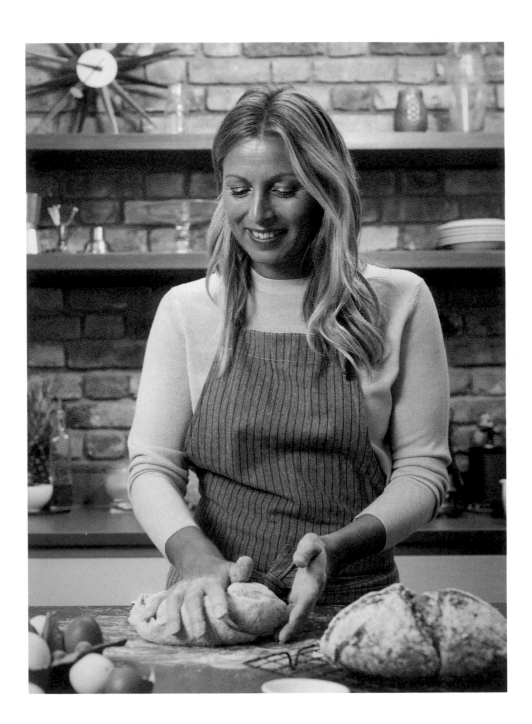

Thank yous

Writing a book during a year or so of lockdowns and restrictions from the COVID pandemic brought on many challenges along the way, so I want to give a massive thanks to each and every one of the amazing team of people involved in getting this book onto the shelves and into our kitchens.

At Quarto Publishing, I'm super grateful to you all, right the way through from commissioning, design, editing, proof reading, indexing, production, publicity, sales and marketing, with specific thanks to Jessica Axe, Charlotte Frost, Melissa Hookway, Izzy Eeles, Sarah Pyke, Liz Somers and Lewis Laney. A big thanks also to Enya Todd for the stunning front cover illustration.

Doing the photoshoot is always the fun part of creating a cookbook, that I really look forward to. Malou Burger, it was an absolute joy to work with you again, you've created a book packed with awesome shots. Thanks also to Lawrence Cannings for assisting you, but more importantly, for eating so many of the bakes. It made packing up at the end of each day take far less time! Becci Woods, you were a star. You styled each and every shot with such wonderful props and creativity, and always had a smile on your face. Cat Byers, you were fantastic to work with. Thanks for keeping on top of all the food prep and copious amounts of baking.

As always, a big thanks to my lovely agent Borra and the team at DML.

I'd like to thank my wonderful family, friends and numerous neighbours who were my chief taste testers during the recipe testing process. Your comments and constructive criticism has been invaluable, and once again I'm sorry for any expanded waistlines!

A heartfelt thanks to both my wonderful grandmothers and my mum, who between them kicked off my love of baking from a very young age and didn't ever complain about the mess I created in their kitchens! I hope all I learned from you continues down our family line.

A final thank you to you to every one of you who choose to cook from *The Flexible Baker*. I hope you enjoy every recipe as much as I do. Happy flexible baking!

www.jo-pratt.com   @cookwithjopratt

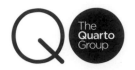

Brimming with creative inspiration, how-to
projects, and useful information to enrich your
everyday life, quarto.com is a favourite destination
for those pursuing their interests and passions.

© 2022 The Quarto Group
Text © 2022 Jo Pratt
Photography © 2022 Malou Burger Photography Limited

First published in 2022 by White Lion Publishing,
an imprint of The Quarto Group.
The Old Brewery, 6 Blundell Street
London, N7 9BH,
United Kingdom

T (0)20 7700 6700
www.QuartoKnows.com

A catalogue record for this book is available from the British Library.

ISBN 978 0 7112 6346 8
Ebook ISBN 978 0 7112 6347 5
10 9 8 7 6 5 4 3 2 1

Assistant food stylist	Cat Byers
Designer	Sarah Pyke
Editor	Charlotte Frost
Photographer's assistant	Laurence Cannings
Props stylist	Rebecca Woods
Publisher	Jessica Axe

Cover illustration by Enya Todd

Printed in China

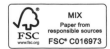